Giving a Voice to those Living with Locked-In Syndrome

Giving a Voice to those Living with Locked-In Syndrome is a unique book that provides a way for the life experiences of people living with Locked-In Syndrome (LiS) to be heard. It combines the personal experiences of those living locked-in, with the biomedical aspects of LiS, including how it is diagnosed and treated, and the technology, such as eye-tracking devices and brain/computer interfaces, enabling those living with LiS to communicate.

By highlighting both the positive and the negative elements of living with LiS, the book aims to encourage change, wherever it is needed in the field of LiS, to guide future diagnostic techniques and enable better, compassionate and appropriate care. Most importantly the book focuses on the moving autobiographies of people living locked-in. These personal accounts show their lives before becoming locked-in; their experiences during the illness or accident that resulted in LiS; how they came to terms mentally, emotionally and physically with their complete change in lifestyle; how those around them, their partners, family, friends and colleagues, adjusted; what is helpful to them and what is frustrating; and finally, their hopes for the future. Autobiographies are drawn from authors all over the globe, allowing readers insights into how LiS is dealt with in different countries, in terms of treatment, care and funding.

It is valuable reading for all professionals working in the brain injury field, including neuropsychologists and those in the caring professions, as well as students in these fields. It will also be relevant for IT students and those working with new technologies.

Shannan Keen has a BA in Psychology and Philosophy, and a Neuroscience Masters from the Brain and Mind Research Institute, University of Sydney. In 2012, as part of her PhD, she founded, and continues to run, the Australian Register for Disorders of Consciousness (ARDoC) within the Brain Foundation. In 2022 she established the annual International Locked-in Syndrome Conference. In 2023 she launched the worldwide Locked-in Syndrome Community Forum on Facebook.

Giving a Voice to those Living with Locked-In Syndrome

Sharing Feelings, Experiences, Hopes and Expectations

Edited by Shannan Keen

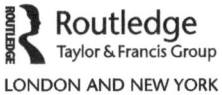

Routledge
Taylor & Francis Group

LONDON AND NEW YORK

Designed cover image: Monique Udo

First published 2025
by Routledge
4 Park Square, Milton Park, Abingdon, Oxon OX14 4RN

and by Routledge
605 Third Avenue, New York, NY 10158

Routledge is an imprint of the Taylor & Francis Group, an informa business

British Library Cataloguing-in-Publication Data
A catalogue record for this book is available from the British Library

ISBN: 9781032734354 (hbk)
ISBN: 9781032733531 (pbk)
ISBN: 9781003464181 (ebk)

DOI: 10.4324/9781003464181

Typeset in Times New Roman
by KnowledgeWorks Global Ltd.

Contents

Contributors

Please Note

Please note that the text in each of the chapters written by the Locked-In Syndrome authors appears exactly as they have provided it. Their choice of repetition or quirky punctuation might not be strictly 'correct' however, since these authors have no form of communicating apart from through their typed words, it is vital that their exact voices are preserved.

List of Authors

Duncan R. Campling; United States
Learn about my journey back from two brainstem strokes a week apart, as a British expat living in Philadelphia.

Dawn Faizey Webster; United Kingdom
I was an IT teacher at a local private grammar school, however, since becoming locked-in I have gained a BA in history, an MA in history of art and am in the final stages of my PhD. I have written a book about my experiences and was involved with Tracey Gibb and Shannan Keen in arranging the first International webinar on LiS.

Bram Harrison; United Kingdom
There are different ways Locked-in Syndrome can quite literally change a life; my case is an acquired brain injury. In 1998, my diagnosis of the condition carried very little information. I hope people today who encounter the condition are better informed. I hope my difficult experiences help make positive decisions.

Ann Johnson; Canada
More than anything I wanted to have kids and a family. Just as I reached my goal, the Brainstem Stroke took it all away.

Bex Kemp; United Kingdom
I was just your average happy 32-year-old who had a massive brainstem stroke and ended up with locked-in syndrome.

Nelleke Koeners (Tars' story); Belgium
I am a child, a woman, a mother trying to juggle all the demands of life. Life has taught me that humor is the best fertilizer for the garden, and therefore, for life. Life has also taught me to take things day by day, which simplifies my life.

Isabelle Lauberthe; France
When my life was all mapped out, how could I have imagined that a piece of cheese would devastate everything in its path?

Julio Lopes Ribeiro; France
I am optimistic, a fighter. I take life as it comes, despite LiS.

Wenche Loseth; Norway
Wenche has given many talks across Norway about living with Locked-in Syndrome. She has also written a book about her struggle to reach the life she lives today. Wenche has her own website, wencheloseth.no, where you can see all the beautiful paintings she creates using her mouth.

Bénédicte Jullien; Belgium
I am recently divorced, living alone and part-time with my two children. I fight daily against the injustices of my country for this pathology.

Dick van der Heijde; The Netherlands
How I am living with Locked-in Syndrome for already 33 years without being bored for a single hour.

Paqui Villegas; Spain
I am a woman with a lot of strength, with courage, with a great desire to improve and a very positive mindset. I am extremely sociable and outgoing and I have a very good heart.

Cover Artist

Monique Udo; Amsterdam
Monique Udo studied saxophone at Sweelinck Conservatory Amsterdam. She has performed contemporary music with the Syrinx Saxophone Quartet. As a music educator, she worked as a saxophone teacher for Musicschool Amsterdam and initiated music education projects in India and Africa. Monique will also be remembered as founder of Muziek Voor Kinderen (Music for Children) a non-profit organization which from 2009 onward supports available and inclusive music education. Amongst which in Uganda her life and even during her illness she never lost her love for drawing.

Professional Contributors

James M. Brinton, CCC-SLP; United States

I am a speech-language pathologist who has worked with children and adults in schools, vocational placements, home-health, rehabilitation hospitals and hospice settings to provide communication assessments, treatments and education. I currently work for Patrona Corporation in Washington, DC, USA, as an assistive technology specialist.

Mohammad Hossein Khosravi; Belgium

Mohammad Hossein Khosravi is a medical doctor and PhD candidate at the University of Liège, Belgium, under the supervision of Professor Steven Laureys. Khosravi focuses on clinical and applied neuroscience, contributing to brain injury research with an emphasis on traumatic brain injuries and neuromodulation.

Steven Laureys; Canada & Belgium

Steven Laureys, MD, PhD, is a neurologist renowned for his expertise on consciousness and cognition, neuroplasticity and neuromodulation. He currently is Chairholder of the Canada Excellence Research Chair in Neuroplasticity, Université Laval, and Invited Professor at Harvard Medical School. He is Chief Neurologist of TRAINM NeuroRehab and BRAIN-NM NeuroModulation Clinics, Antwerp and Amsterdam.

David Moses; United States

David Moses is affiliated with the Department of Neurological Surgery, University of California, San Francisco, San Francisco, California, USA, and the Weill Institute for Neuroscience, University of California, San Francisco, San Francisco, California, USA. He is an adjunct professor at UCSF who, for the last 10+ years, has been working on methods to translate brain signals from a person into what that person was trying to say. His goal is to combine various engineering disciplines, software development, and artificial intelligence to create advanced neurotechnology that restores a voice to persons with Locked-in Syndrome.

Preface

Shannan Keen

Since my University days in Neuroscience, I continue to strive to make a difference to the lives of people who are living with Locked-in Syndrome. In all those years of scientific work, research, collaborations, study and travel, I have witnessed so many acts of dedication, creativity, hard work and kindness. Wherever we come from, whatever our race or culture, able-bodied or having a disability, when we are person-to-person, we want to be good to one another. Diligence and innovation push forward the boundaries of science and medical practices. Kindness and compassion towards others make our lives meaningful.

The contributing authors in this book demonstrate these qualities. Medical professionals, such as Professor Steven Laureys and Dr Mohammad Hossein Khosravi, dedicate their lives to finding ways to diagnose and treat those with LiS. Technical professionals, like Associate Professor David Moses and his colleagues, work tirelessly to bring technologies of brain-computer interfaces (BCI) and Artificial Intelligence (AI) into improving the lives of those who are trapped in silence within their own bodies. Clever, caring inventors, for example James M. Brinton, create and develop devices to enable those living with Locked-in Syndrome to communicate. These people, and many like them the world over, are transforming the lives, abilities, achievements and expectations of those who live Locked-in. This book enables readers, neuroscientists, researchers, medical personnel, carers, family members and people living with LiS to learn from experts working in this field.

Most importantly, the following chapters allow us to gain deep insight into the lives, aims and achievements of these people with LiS. Patience, acceptance, courage, grit, determination, joy and appreciation all contribute to the lives of those struck by accident, illness or stroke. Being given an insight into the coping mechanisms required to move forward with one's life when suddenly profoundly paralysed, only able to blink or move an eye, is confronting, humbling and inspiring.

This book not only recognises and applauds outstanding professional people and their ceaseless work, it is a tribute to twelve of those living Locked-in, each of whom lead meaningful and valued lives. These richly individual accounts show the variety of ways in which they adjusted and coped with the enormous challenges that LiS brings. Their writing is enlightening, inspiring, heart-wrenching and heart-warming. Giving a voice to those who can no longer speak is one of the driving forces for getting this book published.

I encourage you to read and share this book with friends, students and colleagues to enlighten others about this condition.

1 An Introduction to Locked-in-Syndrome: Diagnosis, Care, and Outcomes

Steven Laureys[i,] and Mohammad Hossein Khosravi[ii,iii]*

Note: This introductory chapter is centered around studies conducted by Prof. Steven Laureys and colleagues, while updated data from the literature and recent contributions in the field of Locked-In Syndrome (LIS) were also assessed.

What Is Locked-In-Syndrome and How Does It Affect Patients?

Locked in their bodies, patients with classic Locked-In Syndrome (LIS) suffer from tetraplegia and anarthria while being completely conscious and having intact cognitive function.[1,2] Their motor function is limited to vertical eye movements, which are even absent in patients with complete LIS.[1]

Determining the incidence rate and prevalence of LIS is complicated by its low frequency and diagnostic difficulties. LIS is regarded as exceedingly rare, with only a small number of reported new cases each year. Dutch nursing homes hosted 0.7 patients with classic LIS per 10,000 in 2013, and an estimation reports a prevalence of 0.73 per 100,000 inhabitants in the Netherlands.[3,4] According to the Association du Locked-In Syndrome (ALIS), there are currently over 500 people living with LIS in France.[5] There may be many more cases that go unrecognized or incorrectly diagnosed, suggesting the true incidence may be greater than stated.

Both genders appear to be affected at the same rate, however, some research indicates a slight predominance in males.[6] LIS usually occurs between the third and fifth decades of life, although there are reports of cases in children and patients as old as 77 years of age.[7]

The notion of LIS had been brought up by non-scientific literature long before scientific counterparts, including Émile Zola's novel *Therese Raquin* (Zola, 1979, original 1868) in which he describes a woman trapped alive in a dead body who can only communicate through her eyes.[8] Plum and Posner proposed the first scientific description of LIS in 1972, as inability to move due to quadriplegia with preserved eyelid and vertical eye movements as

DOI: 10.4324/9781003464181-1

well as intact cognitive abilities.[2] Each LIS patient might have a different presentation from others, and that is why Bauer et al. introduced various categories of LIS.[1] Patients with classical LIS suffer from the motor problems described by Plum and Posner. Complete LIS patients have no abilities for any voluntary movements, while those with incomplete LIS have motor capacities above classical LIS, which might represent a transitory stage of recovery.[9]

The most common cause of LIS is bilateral vascular (ischemic or hemorrhagic), lesions of ventral pons, including aneurysm,[10] basilar artery dissection,[11] vasospasm[12] or malformation,[13] and basilar migraine.[14] However, it may occur resulting from a wide range of non-vascular etiologies (e.g., traumatic brain injury[15,16] or multiple sclerosis[17]) or even iatrogenic causes like lumbar puncture.[18] Although the brain stem and ventral pons are the initial locations of the damage, other parts of the brain, such as cortical areas or supra- and infratentorial white matter fibers, might be also affected, consequently.[19,20]

Diagnosing Locked-In-Syndrome

Diagnosing the condition may take weeks, and family members at the bedside are often the first to notice the patient's eye movements. In addition, there are a variety of differential diagnoses for LIS that make a timely and correct diagnosis challenging. Minimally conscious state (MCS), unresponsive wakefulness syndrome (UWS), akinetic mutism, and cognitive motor dissociation (CMD) are the most important ones.[9,21,22] Thus, LIS might be misdiagnosed as a disorder of consciousness (DoC) in case of no clinical suspicion toward it or lack of proper clinical examination. Coma Recovery Scale-Revised (CRS-R) is a behavioral scale used as a gold standard to distinguish UWS and MCS patients based on their behavioral responses.[23] Consequently, CRS-R barely detects consciousness in conscious patients without behavioral outputs due to either paralysis or lack of motivation. This diagnostic challenge might be addressed either by serial bedside evaluations or, more effectively, through complementary paraclinical evaluations. These ancillary evaluations would be of specific benefit for patients with complete LIS who cannot present any eye movements, even if assessment of vertical eye movements is not missed during clinical examinations.[8,24,25]

Brainstem lesions, which are localized using structural MRI, confirm a clinical suspicion of LIS; however, these standard neuroimaging techniques are not able to provide information upon possible functional impairments caused by these lesions. Despite reports of impaired consciousness and cognitive functions in some patients with LIS,[26,27] task-based or functional neuroimaging modalities for detecting consciousness can help with proper diagnosis in the majority of the cases. Event-related paradigms of EEG or fMRI have been previously used for diagnosing LIS.[28]

Eventually, it seems that a multi-modal approach together with LIS-specific bedside evaluation is needed to properly diagnose patients with LIS and differentiate them from patients with disorders of consciousness.[24]

Clinical Care and Rehabilitation of Patients with Locked-In-Syndrome

Upon conquering diagnostic challenges, it comes to overcoming passive approaches of care, as approximately half of the patients were not receiving any kinds of treatment according to a precedent study on French patients.[29] This is also projected from a paucity of original studies on the efficacy of rehabilitation in patients with LIS.

There are studies underlining that a discrepancy in the perception of LIS patients and their caregivers or medical professionals exists.[30,31] Many clinicians commonly think that LIS patients suffer unbearably, with some even suggesting that a life in this condition is even worse than being in a vegetative state.[30,31] At variance with this assumption, most patients adapt to their condition following passing through the initial period of condition, and report a meaningful quality of life.[30,31] These findings give reason to believe that, in fact, the condition as perceived by healthcare professionals is quite different from what patients face. Precedent evidence reveals that these biased healthcare providers consider less-aggressive therapeutic options in patients with LIS.[32]

Moreover, studies which have targeted quality of life in LIS patients reported that a notable proportion of low quality of life scores are rooted in motor impairment.[33] Thus, apart from psychological support, cognitive deficit rehabilitations and medical therapy, patients might benefit from early intensive motor rehabilitation, which boosts functional outcome and reduces the mortality rate.[9,34] In a systematic review on long-term management and prognosis of LIS, authors have pointed to "multidisciplinary rehabilitation" as the foundation of LIS treatment, and the necessity of rapid aggressive physical rehabilitation in sub-acute settings.[33] Robot-assisted gait and upper extremity training have also been effective in previous studies in terms of improving independence, accuracy of upper limb movements, and lower limb function.

Rehabilitation is a crucial determinant of the quality of life of a patient. While little improvement has been noticed in communication and motor recovery among many patients, even modest improvement in such domains did translate to gains in emotional recovery. Studies advocate for focusing the rehabilitation on the patients' ability to partially control their world; implanting a brain-computer interface or improving access to assistive communication equipment would surely accomplish this.[30] Enabling this will allow patients to truly interact with the world and improves their quality of life.[30,31]

Quality of Life of Patients and Caregivers

Assessing the quality of life (QoL) in patients with LIS presents unique challenges, as it involves measuring subjective experiences in individuals who retain cognitive function but experience near-total physical paralysis.[30] Despite these profound limitations, studies have provided a more nuanced understanding of their well-being.

A survey involving 65 chronic LIS patients from the French Association for LIS revealed that 72% of the patients reported feelings of happiness, with a median score of +3 on the Anamnestic Comparative Self-Assessment (ACSA) scale, where +5 represented the best period of their life prior to LIS and -5 the worst.[30] Only 28% of the patients reported unhappiness, with their dissatisfaction often linked to poor mobility, lack of recreational activities, and incomplete recovery of speech. Notably, the study found that a longer duration in the LIS state was associated with greater happiness, suggesting that many patients can adapt to their condition over time.[30] Anxiety and the lack of recovery in speech production were significantly associated with unhappiness, while a shorter duration in LIS emerged as another key factor contributing to emotional distress.[30]

Also another survey that was conducted in 2007 and involved over 80 patients from the French Association for LIS, revealed similar findings.[31] This study reported that 60% of patients were dissatisfied with their mobility and 40% desired more social engagement; however, more than 90% expressed satisfaction with how their activities of daily living needs were met. In addition, over 80% of LIS patients felt that they had meaningful roles to play in their lives and families. In other words, they found purposes and satisfaction for themselves despite the limitations imposed on such roles by physical disability.[31] Most patients also reported a good mental state, with 80% of them never or rarely depressed and only a few having considered suicide, indicating their great mental toughness.

The studies indicate that community reintegration and the ability to participate in recreational activities are significant areas of dissatisfaction among patients with LIS. For instance, the 2011 survey revealed that only 21% of patients engaged in activities they deemed important, while 39% reported severe restrictions in their mobility within the community.[30] These findings highlight the necessity of addressing mobility limitations and creating opportunities for social and recreational engagement to enhance overall quality of life (QoL).

In addition to physical and social limitations, emotional well-being is also a crucial factor. Anxiety was a prevalent issue among those reporting dissatisfaction, and patients with elevated anxiety levels were less likely to experience positive QoL outcomes.[30] The studies underscore the importance of anxiolytic therapy and psychological support to alleviate these emotional burdens. Addressing mental health concerns could significantly enhance the overall well-being of LIS patients.

Although physically disabled, the QoL of patients with LIS is often more positive than generally thought. Most patients learn to cope with their condition over time and lead quite meaningful and fulfilling lives. General happiness tends to correlate highly with community participation, mobility, and emotional support, all of which can be facilitated in targeted healthcare interventions. These findings stand against the common views about LIS and point out the importance of considering the lives of patients as complex, dynamic, and not at all fixed by physical disability.

Despite the significant burden they endure, the needs and effect on the psychological well-being of families of patients with LIS have been minimally investigated.[35] Family and caregivers are regularly in unique situations. Patients will frequently have substantial daily care and support needs, which can lend itself to feelings of psychological and emotional burden. In the initial assessment of their needs, psychological state, and quality of life of relatives, researchers wanted to gain a better understanding of the toll caregiving takes on the feeling of well-being.[35]

Relatives of patients with LIS, particularly, appear to experience a much lower quality of life than average.[35] Additionally, the burden of family caregivers negatively impacted the caregiver's quality of life. The study showed that relatives experience anxiety and depressive thoughts, but the unmet needs for emotional support lend itself to feelings of distress. Specifically, the most important need for caregivers was accessing health information, as more than half of caregivers expressed satisfaction receiving handover information on the patient's condition. However, a little more than half informed that their need for emotional support was significantly unmet, thus negatively affecting the caregiver's quality of life.[35] Family and caregivers generally consider the needs of the patient before their own, thus causing emotional distress. Addressing unmet needs for family caregivers for emotional support and health information can improve family caregivers' quality of life.[35]

Prognosis and Outcome of Patients with Locked-In-Syndrome

The prognosis for LIS is quite varied depending on the cause of the condition. Patients with vascular causes, like cerebrovascular accidents involving the brainstem, usually have limited motor improvement, although some instances of remarkable recovery have been reported.[36–39] On the other hand, nonvascular cases, for instance traumatic ones, generally offer a better prognosis for recovery.

Although a mortality rate of 60 to 75% has been reported for patients in the acute phase of LIS, patients who move on from the acute phase have a 10-year survival rate of 83%.[39,40] In parallel with progresses in healthcare strategies and emergence of new technologies, patients with LIS may have higher life expectancies.[9] Whereas an earlier age at onset significantly correlates with better survival rates, no significant relation exists between the age and overall survival time.[8]

Early rehabilitative care significantly improves outcomes, according to studies in Italian and German rehabilitation centers.[8,34] Early interventions have indeed been associated with improved functional outcomes and reduced mortality rates.[8] Many patients learn to cope with their LIS and may lead relatively normal lives, considering the support of rehabilitation technologies and social support.[8] For example, 44% of the patients with LIS live at home, and many have partial motor recovery, such as slight head, limb, or speech movements. About 50% of patients recover some speech; however, in some cases, this may be limited to single words.[8]

End of Life Decision and Ethics of Life Sustaining

Although requests for euthanasia or the withdrawal of life-sustaining treatment occur, they are uncommon. In the 2011 survey, 7% of patients desired euthanasia, while 58% did not wish to be resuscitated in case of cardiac arrest.[30] These findings indicate the complex emotional dilemmas patients are often placed in, where they have severe physical disabilities and, therefore, a desire to end their lives, yet generally find their lives were worth living after a period of adjustment.[30] It highlights how end-of-life decisions should be approached with patience and sensitivity, allowing the patient adequate time to adapt to their new reality prior to making irreversible choices.[30]

A European survey further examined attitudes toward pain management and end-of-life issues in individuals with LIS. Interestingly, while 74% of the respondents disagreed about treatment withdrawal for patients with LIS, 56% reported they would not wish to be kept alive themselves if they were in that condition.[41] This divergence between general and personal preferences brings out the complexity in making ethical decisions related to LIS.[41]

In addition, approval for the withdrawal of treatment was significantly higher for non-religious respondents and those from Northern Europe, while religious respondents and those from Southern Europe were more likely to oppose it.[41] The study also indicated that some professionals recognize patient autonomy as paramount in such decisions, and for this reason, patients with LIS, because cognitively intact, are competent to make their own decisions regarding the use of life-sustaining treatment or even physician-assisted death. Withdrawing care from conscious patients, despite their physical limitations, is nevertheless a practically universally ethically and legally problematic solution.[41]

A more recent Chinese survey among medical and legal professionals as well as family members provides interesting insights into the fact that 70% of respondents opposed cessation of life-supporting measures for LIS patients.[42] Younger patients (20–30 years of age) and neurologists were more resistant to treatment withdrawal, whereas older respondents considered this more acceptable. It also emerged that 59% of the participants in the survey wanted to continue alive in a chronic state of LIS, though older respondents were more willing to refuse treatment. Moreover, religious orientation had a great influence on such a preference, and religiously oriented respondents were more likely to want to continue being treated.[42]

These findings point to the importance of taking account of individual characteristics and cultural contexts in making ethical decisions on behalf of LIS patients.[42] Further research is needed to delve deeper into the perspectives of the religious community and to respond better to the needs of caregivers to lighten their emotional and practical loads.[42]

In short, this means that patient autonomy is essential for ethical responses in end-of-life care.[41,42] Since LIS patients still preserve the capacity of declaring their wishes, it is of utmost importance to respect them by creating close collaboration among health professionals and family members. Moreover, emotional and medical support should be provided in sufficient amounts. Apart from that, clinicians should refrain from making the decision of early withdrawal-particularly during the acute phases of the syndrome when the patients are still getting acquainted with their new state and do not receive rehabilitation processes yet.[41,42]

Prospects for LIS

While many patients do not regain significant motor function, ongoing research aims to understand better the factors that contribute to improved outcomes.[9] The future for patients with LIS is being shaped by breakthroughs in technology, rehabilitation methods, and a growing understanding of their quality of life. Improvement of communicative and rehabilitative approaches constitutes one of the most relevant research areas for patients with LIS, with the focus being placed on enhancing their quality of life by means of innovative technologies.

Over the years, brain-computer interface technology has improved the lives of LIS patients by providing a very important tool for communication and control.[32] These systems allow LIS patients to communicate independently from muscular input.[43] By means of camera-guided systems tracking eye movements or infrared sensors coupled to virtual keyboards displayed on screens, patients may initiate conversation and control their environment. The BCI has also been used to communicate, surf the Web, and even paint in an artistic manner.[44–49] BCI-controlled devices further provide autonomy to LIS patients in the use of electronic devices, such as lights, wheelchairs, and other environmental controls.

Currently, implantable BCIs focus on translating brain signals related to intended movements into communication commands, therefore offering a direct channel for communication in patients suffering from LIS.[50] It has been shown that BCIs can efficiently detect neural activities, thus allowing users to drive devices simply by thinking.[51]

Future developments will lead to further multichannel inputs-speech, muscle movements, and brain activity-whole input schemes that will vastly expand these systems' capabilities in enabling the person to better interact with the world.

Increasing awareness of capabilities and needs of LIS patients is very essential for helping advance their care and integrate them into society. While LIS is a quite serious disability, advances in technology and supportive models of care, besides a better comprehension of what these patients go through, is offering a more promising outlook for the future. Improvement in their options of communication and rehabilitation processes are vital portions in helping them achieve fulfilled lives despite their disabilities.

What to Expect in the Following Chapters

As this introductory chapter ends, we wish to present a glance at the chapters that will follow. This book explores different aspects of living with LIS in the context of technology and personal experiences.

One chapter will introduce eye-tracking, a technology that has revolutionized communication possibilities for people with LIS. This chapter will explain how eye-tracking works, the ways that it was developed and how it has benefited people who cannot communicate through traditional routes in terms of their potential to improve quality of life. Another chapter will describe BCIs and speech synthesizers. BCIs offer new possibilities for people with LIS to engage with the outside world through using their brain signals. The combination of speech synthesizer technology opens substantial avenues for restoring people to communicate, live more independently, and have more agency in their lives.

However, the core of this book will consist of the twelve autobiographical chapters. Each of these autobiographical chapters will share the personal account from a remarkable individual living with LIS. The personal stories will detail the individual's life prior to developing LIS, and the early experiences they had during and following developing LIS. These accounts intend to articulate many of the emotional, psychological, and social aspects of living with LIS, and the courage required in those aspects which separate these individuals from others.

This convergence between the cutting-edge technology and the emotional and psychological experiences faced is intended to provide a more rounded perspective of the advancements of technology with research concerning human experiences living with LIS.

Declaration of Generative AI in Scientific Writing

During the preparation of this work, the authors used editGPT as a linguistic assistant to improve readability. After using this tool, the authors reviewed and edited the content as needed to make sure of the accuracy and scientific integrity of the text. Moreover, ChatGPT, SciSpace, and Perplexity were used as information search assistants, in addition to conventional keyword-based bibliographic databases, to enhance retrieval of related literature.

Notes

i Chairholder of the Canada Excellence Research Chair in Neuroplasticity Université Laval and Invited Professor at Harvard Medical School. He is Chief Neurologist of TRAINM NeuroRehab and BRAIN-NM NeuroModulation Clinics, Antwerp and Amsterdam.

ii Coma Science Group, GIGA Consciousness, University of Liège, 4000 Liège, Belgium.

iii Centre du Cerveau², University Hospital of Liège, 4000 Liège, Belgium.

* Correspondence to Prof. Steven Laureys.

References

1. Bauer G, Gerstenbrand F, Rumpl E. Varieties of the locked-in syndrome. Journal of Neurology. 1979;221:77–91.
2. Plum F PJ. The diagnosis of stupor and coma. Contemp Neurol Ser. 1972;10: 1–286.
3. Pels EGM, Aarnoutse EJ, Ramsey NF, Vansteensel MJ. Estimated prevalence of the target population for brain-computer interface neurotechnology in the Netherlands. Neurorehabilitation and Neural Repair. 2017;31(7):677–85.
4. Kohnen R, Lavrijsen J, Bor J, Koopmans R. The prevalence and characteristics of patients with classic locked-in syndrome in Dutch nursing homes. Journal of Neurology. 2013;260:1527–1534.
5. Association du Locked-in Syndrome (ALIS). Qu'est-ce que le Locked-In Syndrome? https://alis-asso.fr/quest-ce-que-le-lis/
6. Das JM AK, Asuncion RMD. Locked-in syndrome. [Updated 2023 Jul 24]. In: StatPearls [Internet]. Treasure Island (FL): StatPearls Publishing; 2024 Jan.
7. León-Carrión J, van Eeckhout P, Domínguez-Morales Mdel R, Pérez-Santamaría FJ. The locked-in syndrome: a syndrome looking for a therapy. Brain Inj. 2002; 16(7):571–582.
8. Laureys S, Pellas F, Van Eeckhout P, Ghorbel S, Schnakers C, Perrin F, et al. The locked-in syndrome: what is it like to be conscious but paralyzed and voiceless? Progress in Brain Research. 2005;150:495–611.
9. Schnetzer L, McCoy M, Bergmann J, Kunz A, Leis S, Trinka E. Locked-in syndrome revisited. Therapeutic Advances in Neurological Disorders. 2023;16: 17562864231160873.
10. Kolić Z, Kukuljan M, Vukas D, Bonifačić D, Vrbanec K, Franić IK. Locked-in syndrome in a patient with acute obstructive hydrocephalus, caused by large unruptured aneurysm of the basilar artery (BA). British Journal of Neurosurgery. 2017;31(6):738–740.
11. Inatomi Y, Nakajima M, Yonahara T. Transient total locked-in syndrome due to vertebral and basilar artery dissection. BMJ Case Reports CP. 2021;14(2):e238912.
12. Lacroix G, Couret D, Combaz X, Prunet B, Girard N, Bruder N. Transient locked-in syndrome and basilar artery vasospasm. Neurocritical Care. 2012;16:145–147.

13. Maramattom BV, Bhattacharjee S. Decerebrate rigidity with preservation of consciousness in pontine hemorrhage with complete neurologic recovery. Neurology India. 2019;67(3):881.
14. Sulkava R, Kovanen J. Locked-in syndrome with rapid recovery: a manifestation of basilar artery migraine? Headache: The Journal of Head and Face Pain. 1983;23(5):238–239.
15. Tung RC, Vivar-Cruz PW. Locked-in syndrome. Kansas Journal of Medicine. 2019;12(2):56.
16. Kartum T, Baş G, Kemerdere R, Hanci M. Posttraumatic locked-in syndrome from combined brainstem and upper cervical injury in childhood: a case report. Neurochirurgie. 2022;68(6):e104–e6.
17. Keme-Ebi IK, Asindi AA. Locked-in syndrome in a Nigerian male with multiple sclerosis: a case report and literature review. Pan African Medical Journal. 2008;1(1).
18. Chen JA, Driver J, Segar D, Bernstock JD, Gupta S, Gormley W. Medullary infarction leading to locked-in syndrome following lumbar puncture in a patient with basilar invagination. World Neurosurgery. 2020;137:292–295.
19. Leonard M, Renard F, Harsan L, Pottecher J, Braun M, Schneider F, et al. Diffusion tensor imaging reveals diffuse white matter injuries in locked-in syndrome patients. PLOS One. 2019;14(4):e0213528.
20. Sarà M, Cornia R, Conson M, Carolei A, Sacco S, Pistoia F. Cortical brain changes in patients with locked-in syndrome experiencing hallucinations and delusions. Frontiers in Neurology. 2018;9:354.
21. Claassen J, Kondziella D, Alkhachroum A, Diringer M, Edlow BL, Fins JJ, et al. Cognitive motor dissociation: gap analysis and future directions. Neurocritical Care. 2023:1–18.
22. Laureys S, Owen AM, Schiff ND. Brain function in coma, vegetative state, and related disorders. Lancet Neurol. 2004;3(9):537–546.
23. Giacino JT, Kalmar K, Whyte J. The JFK Coma Recovery Scale-Revised: measurement characteristics and diagnostic utility. Archives of physical medicine and rehabilitation. 2004;85(12):2020–2029.
24. Kondziella D, Bender A, Diserens K, van Erp W, Estraneo A, Formisano R, et al. European Academy of Neurology guideline on the diagnosis of coma and other disorders of consciousness. European Journal of Neurology. 2020;27(5):741–756.
25. Lesenfants D, Habbal D, Chatelle C, Soddu A, Laureys S, Noirhomme Q. Toward an attention-based diagnostic tool for patients with locked-in syndrome. Clin EEG Neurosci. 2018;49(2):122–135.
26. Seidl M, Golaszewski S, Kunz A, Nardone R, Bauer G, Trinka E, Gerstenbrand F. The locked-in plus syndrome. Journal of the Neurological Sciences. 2013;333:e263–e4.
27. Kumral E, Dorukoğlu M, Uzunoğlu C, Çetin FE. The clinical and cognitive spectrum of locked-in syndrome: 1-year follow-up of 100 patients. Acta Neurologica Belgica. 2022;122(1):113–121.
28. Schnakers C, Perrin F, Schabus M, Hustinx R, Majerus S, Moonen G, et al. Detecting consciousness in a total locked-in syndrome: an active event-related paradigm. Neurocase. 2009;15(4):271–277.
29. León-Carrión J, Eeckhout Pv, Dominguez-Morales MDR, Pérez-Santamaría FJ. Survey: the locked-in syndrome: a syndrome looking for a therapy. Brain injury. 2002;16(7):571–582.

30. Bruno M-A, Bernheim JL, Ledoux D, Pellas F, Demertzi A, Laureys S. A survey on self-assessed well-being in a cohort of chronic locked-in syndrome patients: happy majority, miserable minority. BMJ Open. 2011;1(1):e000039.
31. Bruno M.A. PF, Bernheim J.L., Ledoux D., Goldman S., Demertzi A., Majerus S., Vanhaudenhuyse A., et al. Quelle vie après le locked-in syndrome? Rev Med Liege. 2008;63:445–451.
32. Lulé D, Zickler C, Häcker S, Bruno M-A, Demertzi A, Pellas F, et al. Life can be worth living in locked-in syndrome. Progress in Brain Research. 2009;177: 339–351.
33. Halan T, Ortiz JF, Reddy D, Altamimi A, Ajibowo AO, Fabara SP. Locked-in syndrome: a systematic review of long-term management and prognosis. Cureus. 2021;13(7).
34. Casanova E, Lazzari RE, Lotta S, Mazzucchi A. Locked-in syndrome: improvement in the prognosis after an early intensive multidisciplinary rehabilitation. Archives of physical medicine and rehabilitation. 2003;84(6):862–867.
35. Lugo Z, Pellas F, Blandin V, Laureys S, Gosseries O. Assessment of needs, psychological impact and quality of life in families of patients with locked-in syndrome. Brain Inj. 2017;31(12):1590–1596.
36. Patterson JR, Grabois M. Locked-in syndrome: a review of 139 cases. Stroke. 1986;17(4):758–764.
37. McCusker EA, Rudick RA, Honch GW, Griggs RC. Recovery from the 'locked-in' syndrome. Archives of Neurology. 1982;39(3):145–147.
38. Ebinger G, Huyghens L, Corne L, Aelbrecht W. Reversible "locked-in" syndromes. Intensive Care Medicine. 1985;11:218–219.
39. Doble JE, Haig AJ, Anderson C, Katz R. Impairment, activity, participation, life satisfaction, and survival in persons with locked-in syndrome for over a decade: follow-up on a previously reported cohort. The Journal of Head Trauma Rehabilitation. 2003;18(5):435–444.
40. Nikić PM, Jovanović D, Paspalj D, Georgievski-Brkić B, Savić M. Clinical characteristics and outcome in the acute phase of ischemic locked-in syndrome: case series of twenty patients with ischemic LIS. Eur Neurol. 2013;69(4):207–212.
41. Demertzi A, Jox RJ, Racine E, Laureys S. A European survey on attitudes towards pain and end-of-life issues in locked-in syndrome. Brain Injury. 2014;28(9):1209–1215.
42. Yan Y, Demertzi A, Xia Y, Wang J, Hu N, Zhang Z, et al. Ethics of life-sustaining treatment in locked-in syndrome: A Chinese survey. Annals of Physical and Rehabilitation Medicine. 2020;63(6):483–487.
43. Dornhege G. Toward brain-computer interfacing: MIT press; 2007.
44. Birbaumer N, Ghanayim N, Hinterberger T, Iversen I, Kotchoubey B, Kübler A, et al. A spelling device for the paralysed. Nature. 1999;398(6725):297–298.
45. Neumann N, Kübler A, Kaiser J, Hinterberger T, Birbaumer N. Conscious perception of brain states: mental strategies for brain–computer communication. Neuropsychologia. 2003;41(8):1028–1036.
46. Nijboer F, Sellers EW, Mellinger J, Jordan MA, Matuz T, Furdea A, et al. A P300-based brain–computer interface for people with amyotrophic lateral sclerosis. Clinical Neurophysiology. 2008;119(8):1909–1916.
47. Muglerab E, Benschc M, Haldera S, Rosenstielc W, Bogdancd M, Birbaumerae N, Kübleraf A. Control of an internet browser using the P300 event-related potential. International Journal of Bioelectromagnetism. 2008;10(1):56–63.

48. Karim AA, Hinterberger T, Richter J, Mellinger J, Neumann N, Flor H, et al. Neural internet: web surfing with brain potentials for the completely paralyzed. Neurorehabilitation and Neural Repair. 2006;20(4):508–515.

49. Kübler A, Botrel L. The making of brain painting—from the idea to daily life use by people in the locked-in state. Brain Art: Brain-Computer Interfaces for Artistic Expression. 2019:409–431.

50. Müller-Putz G, Crell M, Egger J, Suwandjieff P, Kostoglou K. Towards implantable brain-computer interface for communication in locked-in syndrome patients. An introduction to INTRECOM. 2023;9(2):1–4.

51. Voity K, Lopez T, Chan JP, Greenwald BD. Update on how to approach a patient with locked-in syndrome and their communication ability. Brain Sciences. 2024; 14(1):92.

2 Communication from Gestures to Gadgets

James M. Brinton

Working as a young speech-language pathologist, I was called to visit the hospital room of a woman with multiple systems atrophy to evaluate her communication abilities and introduce tools that she and her husband could use together. The room she lived in, although sterile and plain, was lovingly decorated to create a cozy home-away-from-home feel. While her muscles had atrophied over time, her mind was sharp and her soul was eager to connect with the world. A week before my visit, she had been lent an old communication device that had been dropped off without instruction or support, leaving her without hope. Tears filled her eyes as her husband explained what they had hoped for. They heard that she could use her eye movements to communicate with the right training and tools in place, and her husband explained her recent attempts to operate the old device, without any success.

As I always do, I asked the woman to indicate for me her sign for *"yes"* and sign for *"no"* so I could ask her questions directly. Through miniscule movements of her face and eyes, she was able to answer yes or no as I asked questions to get to know her better. After a quick assessment of her eye function and ability to follow directions, I set up a communication device I had brought—an eye gaze communication system she could operate with her eye movements.

Her eyes looked intently at the yellow calibration points on the screen, and then she was presented with an on-screen keyboard, along with instructions to look at letters, wait for the "click" sound, and spell a word. Never knowing what someone will type first, I waited as she began.

"Click, click, click, click..." her eyes got to work, and I looked over her bedside as her husband quietly waited in the corner of the room. The message she spelled: A-M-A-Z-O-N.

"Amazon?" I exclaimed. With a perplexed glance I looked in her husband's direction, hoping for understanding. His face had lit up with a huge grin and tears began pouring down his cheeks as he explained that she was—*in his words*—a shopaholic, and that she was telling us that she wanted to shop online at www.Amazon.com!

DOI: 10.4324/9781003464181-2

Over my years of practice, I have waited eagerly as locked-in patients spell their first utterances after long delays of having no tools to communicate. These first words often reflect things of the heart. Phrases like, "*I love you,*" "*Happy birthday Honey,*" "*Hello everyone,*" or "*Make sure my son has new school shoes,*" can be common.

In the wisdom gathered over time while waiting for communication to be restored to him, one man carefully spelled an unforgettable life lesson: "*To communicate is to be alive!*" It is evident that humans, from the earliest measurable indicators, are designed to socially connect and communicate with others. An infant's first words are the beginning of a lifetime of communication. Even when the ability to speak stops due to disability, we continue to have this constant desire for connection and social interaction.

When someone becomes locked-in due to accident or a diagnosed condition, they experience communication declines that lead to immense frustration, fear, and isolation. Communication is a shared activity, and the loss of voice not only impacts them, but their shared relationship with family members, caregivers, and friends. Loss of communication can include these experiences:

- Failed attempts to communicate their message
- Abandonment of ideas
- Reduced participation in daily routines
- Decreased sense of connectedness with the world around them
- Increased despair or sadness
- Dependence upon communication partners to interpret communication attempts
- Dependence upon communication partners to anticipate daily wants and needs

Meanwhile the introduction of communication tools and training can allow them to:

- Type and create messages with digitized speech
- Advocate for themselves
- Participate in family decision-making
- Agree or disagree with someone
- Express wants, needs, and desires
- Communicate in emergency situations and episodes of pain
- Direct the behavior of their caregivers
- Engage people in the community
- Work from home by accessing a computer
- Use a telephone, the internet, and communicate by SMS text message
- Participate in online activities like games, support groups, and research
- Nurture family relationships through communication

All People Have the Fundamental Right to Communicate

For the remainder of this chapter, I will speak directly to the readers who can no longer speak on their own. In the United States, The Communication Bill of Rights, created by the National Joint Committee for the Communication Needs of Persons with Severe Disabilities, is a powerful description of your fundamental rights to communicate. It includes:

1 The right to interact socially, maintain social closeness, and build relationships
2 The right to request desired objects, actions, events, and people
3 The right to refuse or reject undesired objects, actions, events, or choices
4 The right to express personal preferences and feelings
5 The right to make choices from meaningful alternatives
6 The right to make comments and share opinions
7 The right to ask for and give information, including information about changes in routine and environment
8 The right to be informed about people and events in your life
9 The right to access interventions and supports that improve communication
10 The right to have communication acts acknowledged and responded to even when the desired outcome cannot be realized
11 The right to always have access to functioning AAC (augmentative and alternative communication) and other AT (assistive technology) services and devices
12 The right to access environmental contexts, interactions, and opportunities that promote participation as full communication partners with other people, including peers
13 The right to be treated with dignity and addressed with respect and courtesy
14 The right to be addressed directly and not be spoken for or talked about in the third person while present
15 The right to have clear, meaningful, and culturally and linguistically appropriate communications.

This resource can be accessed online at https://www.asha.org/njc/communication-bill-of-rights/.

Communication tools from no-tech to high-tech: Augmentative and alternative communication (AAC) methods include any number of tools or gadgets that can *augment* or provide *alternative ways* to get your message across. Some of these require no technology like homemade paper tools, while others are electronic.

Yes/No Communication: Albeit limiting in many ways, finding a simple and reliable way to communicate "yes" and "no" can provide quick access to communication between you and your communication partner. Depending on what part of your body moves a little—it could be a raise of the eyebrow, purse of the lips, smile, or glance—you can decide what small signal you give indicates a "yes" answer, and what different signal indicates "no." Here are a few examples I've seen: Raise the eyebrows up for yes, purse the lips for no. Look right for yes, look left for no. Click the tongue for yes, do not click for no. If these are too difficult, use any small signal you can give to mean "yes" and do nothing to indicate "no." While some people rely on blinking to indicate yes and no, this can be easily complicated due to our eye's natural reflex to blink at any given time.

To communicate with yes/no, have your communication partner ask simple and short yes/no questions, then wait for your signal. Use your established signs to indicate yes or no in response. These questions need to be asked one at a time and should not be convoluted. So instead of, "*Are you cold, or doing ok, or do you want your blanket?*" they should ask, "*Are you cold?*" (wait for response), then "*Do you want your blanket?*" (wait for second response). Have your family teach everyone who visits, including friends and medical staff, your yes/no communication method.

Communication Poster: A large centrally-located poster can be used to quickly scan through the most frequently asked requests you make. Have a simple poster made that lists your frequent needs, with a number assigned to each item. Customize your requests in order of importance. Some examples might include: 1. Suction, 2. Water, 3. Medicine, 4. Adjust pillows, 5. I'm cold, 6. I'm hot, 8. Pain, 9. Glasses, 10. Tissue, 11. Play music, 12. Alphabet board.

Communication device, etc. When you need to make a request using this list, intentionally glance at the poster to indicate that you are requesting something. Your communication partner will carefully say 1, 2, 3, 4, and so on, watching for your signal for "yes" when they read the number of the item you are requesting. This system of communication can be used by anyone who enters the room when you want a quick way to request something, using minimal effort.

Alphabet boards: This tool and communication technique goes by many names, so search online for some of the following resources: Partner-assisted scanning, partner-assisted spelling, letterboard, alphabet board, or A-E-I-O-U board. This shared communication technique takes practice, and requires letter sequencing and memory for you and your communication partner. It can be like learning to dance with a new partner—you are going to step over each other at times, but this can be very effective to communicate specific messages. You can find video examples of partner-assisted scanning online, and these video examples can be a valuable model for practice.

This paper communication tool can be dual-sided and include some of the following items. Side one: Rows of alphabet letters, numbers, Yes/No, and "other side." Side two: Frequent requests (much like the communication poster mentioned above), pain scale from 1–10, as well as simple diagrams of the body to indicate where pain is occurring.

A	B	C	D	SPACE	CATEGORIES – TURN BOARD OVER
E	F	G	H	MISTAKE	START OVER
I	J	K	L	M	N
O	P	Q	R	S	T
U	V	W	X	Y	Z

0	1	2	3	4	5	6	7	8	9	10

An example of a partner-assisted spelling board

As your communication partner slowly points row by row, they can read the row out loud and will watch for you to indicate "yes" when they get to your desired letter's row. For example, they will read "A row, E row, I row, O row, U row, numbers" and watch for your signal. Once the row is identified, they scan horizontally until they arrive at your desired letter and watch for your "yes" signal. Since composing a message in little letters requires a lot of memory, it can be helpful for your communication partner to use a small pad of paper and pencil or white board to jot down words as you spell them, thus decreasing memory demands across the entire message.

With practice, many couples become fluent in using partner-assisted scanning to have detailed conversations. Once you both become comfortable, you may be okay with your communication partner guessing or predicting certain words once you start them, if it makes it easier for increased speed.

E-Tran board: An eye-transfer board is a tool that may be used less than others, but it can provide a strong visual medium between communication partners. It can be made of plexiglass or other rigid, clear material that is shaped like a picture frame. Your communication partner will hold it up between both parties, so you can see each other's eye movement and the items on the E-Tran board. With this setup, you can clearly point, by moving your eyes, to the desired letters or words on the board to communicate messages. To practice this method of communication, it will be helpful to search for video tutorials online that demonstrate E-Tran communication.

Eye gaze communication devices: Since the late 1980s, a handful of companies have carefully crafted and refined eye gaze technology to accommodate individuals who have communication disabilities. These high-tech devices are expensive and require practice, much like learning how to play a new instrument, but can open the world of digital communication and connection for someone who is locked-in without body movement.

An eye gaze device is made of a computer tablet with communication software, an eye-tracking camera that looks at the movement of one or both eyes, and a mount to position the device in front of you. The eye tracker includes an infrared light that pulses invisible light onto the eyes while taking pictures. These constant photographs of your eyes (around 60 frames per second) are digitized and analyzed by the device's software, and create a live video of your eye movement as they look at the screen. The communication software is accessed by simply looking at buttons, icons or letter keys on the screen for a specified period of time to "push" the keys. For example, if you look at the letter "B" for .6 seconds, it would press the letter, and you string letters together to form words. Once you have looked at each letter in the word, you look at the "Speak" key, and the device speaks your typed word using a digital voice.

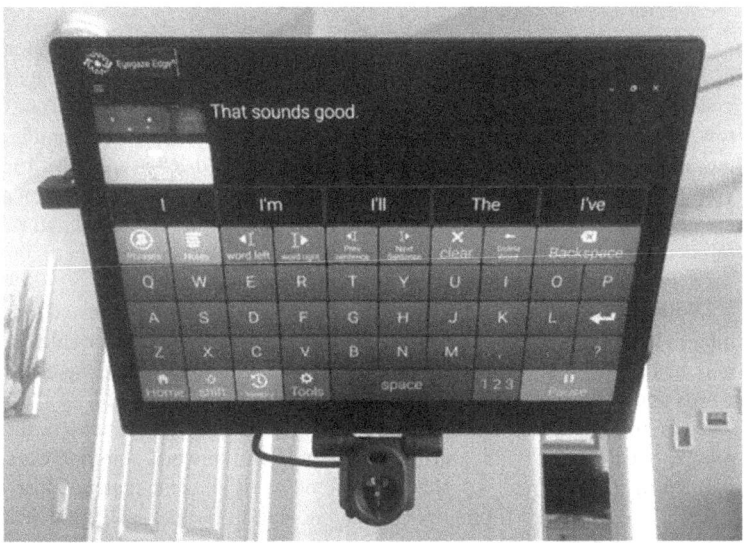

An eye gaze communication device suspended over a person in bed.

These devices use your eye movement to type on a keyboard, move and click a mouse, and access communication pages and computer functions. This includes surfing the internet with your eyes, accessing games, email, and synchronizing with a smart phone for SMS text messaging and calls. Other features include word processing, accessing environmental controls, emergency call bells, and entertainment. The ability to use an eye gaze communication device depends on many physiological and environmental factors, and not everyone's eyes are compatible with these devices. Here are a few questions to ask prior to using a device:

Are you able to move your eyes up, down, left, and right independently? If you have limited eye movement, know that some devices can compensate and accommodate for this. Are you able to use liquid tears (eye drops)? Having hydrated eyes will allow an eye tracker to read your movements accurately. Have you had previous eye surgeries or eye conditions? Mention these to the various manufacturers as you are doing your research, as some devices can accommodate for these better than others. If you have the opportunity to try different devices, you'll want to select the one that provides you the highest accuracy and easiest access. A trained speech-language pathologist can guide you in finding the best tools for you.

Remember that using any of these new communication tools is much like getting on a bicycle for the first time. It will take practice, more practice, and a lot of patience! Celebrate the small successes as they come. For eye gaze communication, obtain a strong calibration and practice large, easy buttons first. Once you are comfortable, move onto smaller buttons and begin spelling words, then phrases, then sentences. When your energy is spent, give yourself a break and use other communication techniques. With these high-tech advancements, there have been individuals who have written blogs and books, earned degrees, composed music, and even continued to work from home. Some well-established manufacturers to research include Eyegaze Inc. (USA), Smartbox (UK), and Tobii Dynavox (USA). Ask each company if they have a process for sending a trial device, how they provide training and support, and how their communication device will accommodate for your unique eyes.

Do you consider yourself a patient person? Great—now double your ability to extend patience and grace as you learn new methods of communication. In spoken language, the average rate of communication for English speaking adults is approximately 150 words per minute. When verbal communication has been lost, and communication tools are put in place, the speed of transmission decreases significantly—even down to 5–15 words per minute. You are required to be diligent, precise, and tremendously patient with your communication partner, and they, even more so, are required to be patient with you.

Your communication partners must become comfortable with added wait time between letters, words, and ideas. Encourage them to keep questions simple and direct, allowing you to take your time. If you or they become impatient or frustrated, you have permission to take a break and try again when ready. Keep in mind that even with these strategies in place, using alternative and augmentative communication is hard work, and can be coupled with big emotions! Using any of these methods shifts responsibility to the communication partner to provide opportunities to communicate, to patiently use the materials, and to verify your message. It is imperative that your communication partner respects and supports your rights and needs to communicate.

In his book, *Shells: Sustained by Grace Within the Tempest,* author Steve Heronemus, who was diagnosed with ALS and typed the book using his eye gaze communication device, summed up his communication experiences beautifully:

"The voice I chose is neither romantic nor Hollywood-esque; it is mechanical and not my own. The machine's pronunciations aren't always accurate. Conversations are slow and I'm often a topic behind. But, through all of this, the people who surround me gently persuaded me that my voice is more about what I say rather than how I sound, that my identity rings more clearly through what comes out from inside my character than in the machine that makes speech possible. My individual voice is still a loss all of my family grieves, but I am beginning to accept that I can make a difference in my world in a different way, finding a voice to spread love, comfort, peace and grace to those around me."

3 Brain-Computer Interfaces and the Future of Assistive Communication

David Moses

Introduction

Locked-in Syndrome (LiS) imposes a multitude of challenges and difficulties upon those who live with it. At the root of some of the most profoundly debilitating of these difficulties is the impairment to natural communication caused by LiS, which leads to drastic reductions in autonomy, self-expression, social presence, and various other aspects of daily life.[1,2] Martin Pistorius, a man who spent many years with LiS without anyone else knowing that he was fully aware of his surroundings, stated: *"I don't know if it's truly possible to express in words what it's like not to be able to communicate. Your personality appears to vanish into a heavy fog and all of your emotions and desires are constricted, stifled and muted within you."*[3]

A major focus of clinicians, scientists, engineers, caregivers, family members, advocates, and patients themselves is to develop methods that restore as much communicative capacity as possible to persons living with LiS. This is primarily done through augmentative and alternative communication (AAC) technology, which is a set of tools and devices that can help persons with LiS express themselves. From picture and letter boards to digital speech-generating devices controlled via eye trackers, a variety of AAC technology exists to support patients with a wide range of communication disorders.[4] Although these tools can be transformative for patients with LiS who would not be able to meaningfully communicate without them, they have several drawbacks compared to natural speech: they are slower, more effortful, less intuitive, require visually attending to a screen or board, and may become unusable if the user loses reliable eye-movement control.[5,6]

Brain-computer interfaces (BCIs) are a promising new form of AAC technology, enabling control over communication interfaces by translating signals recorded from the user's brain into intended text, speech, and other expressive outputs.[7,8] By relying on the user's intent as the control mechanism, BCIs have the potential to restore more naturalistic and effortless communication compared to traditional AAC technology. For example, a patient with LiS could simply try to speak, and a BCI could analyze the patient's brain signals

DOI: 10.4324/9781003464181-3

during the speech attempt and generate the intended speech in an artificial voice. This type of BCI is referred to as a "speech neuroprosthesis,"[9-11] and researchers at multiple institutions have recently made significant advances toward bringing this concept into practical, clinically viable solutions for patients (Figure 3.1).

This chapter focuses on the development of speech neuroprostheses and how they can shape the future of assistive-communication technology. First, the neuroscience of speech processing in the brain is introduced, which guided the early conceptualizations of speech neuroprostheses. Then, an overview of how speech neuroprostheses work is given, followed by descriptions of recent proof-of-concept demonstrations of the technology. Finally, the chapter concludes with expectations for how speech neuroprostheses will fit into the AAC landscape as a restorative option for patients with LiS.

How Speaking Is Represented in the Brain

Speaking is an extraordinarily complex action that involves a neural pathway with many stages, from message conceptualization (the speaker figuring out what meaning or concept they would like to convey to a listener) to acoustic realization (the speaker verbally producing the speech sounds that convey that meaning). Researchers across the globe are still actively pursuing a complete understanding of this neural pathway, but enough progress has been made to inform the feasibility and scientific basis of speech neuroprostheses. This section aims to summarize these findings before going into more detail on how speech neuroprostheses operate.

A brain area called the sensorimotor cortex (SMC) contains neural populations (groups of neurons) that control the rapid, precise, and highly coordinated movements of the vocal tract and enable spoken speech.[10,12-15] These neural populations send commands downstream to neurons in the brainstem and subsequently to neurons that control articulatory muscles in the lips, tongue, jaw, and larynx, orchestrating the movement of these articulators as air is exhaled to produce speech.

Researchers have studied how certain characteristics in the produced speech map to certain activation patterns in the neural populations in the SMC. In the earliest known studies, neurosurgeons directly stimulated SMC sites on the surface of the brain and documented resulting movements and sensations, mapping out how neural populations in the SMC are spatially organized relative to the articulators that they functionally control.[14-16] These findings were largely corroborated by and expanded on in subsequent studies using more sophisticated neural sensors and statistical approaches, characterizing the link between representations of certain properties of spoken speech and vocal-tract control in the SMC.[12,13,17-19] Another set of studies showed that brain activity in the SMC strongly encodes the movement dynamics of the articulators themselves (compared to acoustic properties of the spoken speech).[19,20]

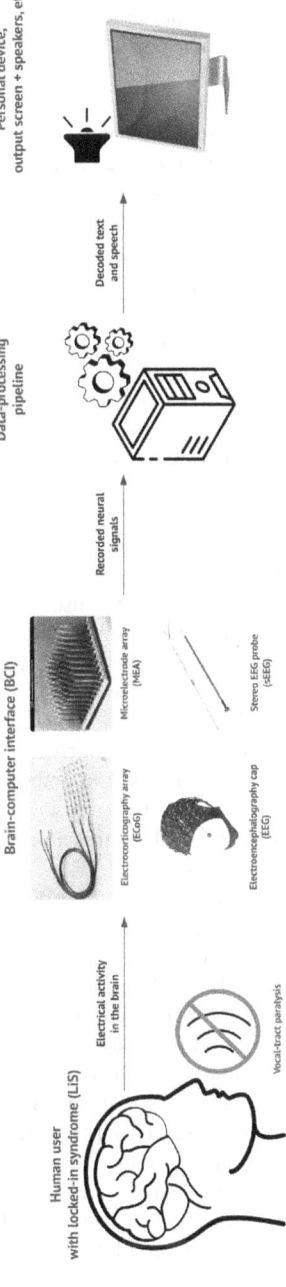

Figure 3.1 Schematic of a speech neuroprosthesis. A human user with locked-in syndrome (LiS), who has vocal-tract paralysis due to LiS, attempts to say something. A brain-computer interface (BCI) records electrical activity from the brain and transfers the signals to a data-processing pipeline. The BCI images show four different recording methodologies for sampling neural signals from the brain. The pipeline processes the neural signals and applies artificial intelligence (AI) models to the signals to decode what the user attempted to say, as text and/or as speech. The decoded output is presented on a personal device or through other hardware. Note that the data-processing pipeline and AI models could be implemented on the personal device instead of on separate hardware. The manufacturers of the BCIs depicted in this figure are as follows: ECoG - PMT Corporation; MEA - Blackrock Neurotech; EEG - Compumedics Neuroscan; sEEG - NeuroOne Medical Technologies Corp.

In summary, a wealth of research exists that describes how brain activity in the SMC controls the vocal tract during speech production. Various characteristics of spoken speech are represented by neural-activation patterns across the SMC, including acoustic aspects of the speech sounds and aspects of the vocal-tract movements that gave rise to those sounds. The studies cited in this section largely investigated how these speech characteristics are "encoded" in neural activity; the next section covers the inverse approach of decoding speech characteristics directly from neural activity, a methodology underlying all speech neuroprostheses.

Decoding Speech from Brain Activity

With the growing knowledge base of how speech is represented in brain activity, an important parallel line of investigation centers around best practices for decoding speech from brain activity. Development of computational approaches for speech decoding is a critical step in creating effective speech neuroprostheses. This section covers early efforts to develop these approaches and how these efforts were enabled by parallel advances in artificial intelligence (AI).

Before describing these computational approaches, it is worth commenting on the different types of hardware used in BCI approaches (Figure 3.1). The vast majority of BCI studies cited in this chapter use "invasive" methodologies, meaning that the interface with the brain requires some level of direct contact with brain tissue. Specifically, these studies primarily use electrocorticography (ECoG), an invasive method which involves placing an array of electrical sensors directly on the surface of the brain without penetrating the brain tissue. Another popular invasive method is microelectrode array (MEA) recording, which involves penetrating brain tissue to embed sensors within the brain, typically near the brain surface. Finally, stereo electroencephalography (sEEG) is an invasive method which involves implanting probes containing electrical sensors deep within brain tissue.

In contrast, "non-invasive" methodologies are those that do not require direct contact with brain tissue. A popular non-invasive BCI method is electroencephalography (EEG), which involves placing electrical sensors on the scalp. The highest-performing speech BCIs all use invasive methods, as the direct contact with brain tissue yields higher-resolution signals, although speech-decoding methods using EEG and other non-invasive recordings are still being actively explored.[21-25] A major tradeoff between the two broad categories of approaches is the increased risk, expense, and complexity of invasive methods caused by the need for surgery to implant the sensors. Before complex studies aimed at assessing the feasibility of speech neuroprostheses with persons with LiS could be fully justified, researchers first pursued successful demonstrations of BCI-based speech decoding with able speakers who had invasive BCI devices implanted as part of their clinical treatment for unrelated diseases (commonly ECoG arrays covering SMC as part of their epilepsy treatment). As a result, the early studies of speech decoding from brain activity cited in this section are all with able speakers, with the expectation that the knowledge gained from these studies would lay the groundwork for speech-neuroprosthetic research with persons with LiS.

As another brief aside, it is helpful to define what is meant by "AI" in the context of speech BCIs. Although AI comes in many forms, here AI is generally used to denote methods for transforming some types of inputs into some types of outputs after first learning a reasonable mapping between the two. For example, to train an AI model for a speech BCI, it is common to have the BCI user first say (or attempt to say) many different words or sentences while their brain activity is recorded, enabling the AI model to subsequently "learn" how specific patterns in the brain activity correspond to specific speech outputs. Once trained, the model can then be used to translate previously unseen brain-activity patterns into speech output, potentially even decoding speech in real time as the user attempts to speak. This is just one type of AI that supports speech-BCI implementations; others will be introduced throughout the remainder of the chapter, with some modeling the statistics of language or the acoustic patterns of spoken speech.

Advances in automatic speech recognition (ASR), an AI-driven field of research that encompasses methods to translate acoustic speech signals into text, have enabled users to speak to devices while the devices interpret what the users say (such as Amazon's Alexa or Apple's Siri). These systems use AI model architectures and language-modeling techniques that decode text from speech acoustics.[26–28] As a fortunate synergy between that field of research and speech-BCI research, researchers discovered that many of the computational approaches from ASR research can also be successfully applied to decoding text from speech-related brain activity (instead of from acoustics).[29] For example, language models that predict the likelihood of possible next words in a sequence given the preceding words—which drive auto-complete features that suggest the next words in a message to users on smartphones, word processors, and email clients—are applicable whether the text is being created from typing, acoustic, or neural inputs.[30]

Two early speech-decoding studies showed that spoken words and sentences could be decoded from ECoG recordings using common ASR techniques.[31,32] Subsequent work showed improved performance using deep-learning ASR methods to decode spoken sentences from ECoG recordings, with one study achieving 90% accuracy with a vocabulary of nearly 2,000 unique words.[33] Another study demonstrated how a text-decoding model for a particular BCI user can be improved by first training the model on data from a separate user, illustrating how incorporating data from multiple users can improve performance for each individual user.[34] These studies show that brain activity can be decoded into text with favorable accuracy, informed by ASR techniques and previous findings of speech representations in the brain.

Although the ability to translate brain activity into text offers significant utility to speech-neuroprosthetic applications, an ideal speech neuroprosthesis would also enable the user to communicate in spoken speech. Speech carries expressive information beyond what is conveyed in text alone, including speaker identity and emphasis.[35] Text-to-speech (TTS) synthesizers are advanced software tools that can synthesize, or generate, naturalistic speech directly from text using AI models.[36–39] TTS synthesizers can be found in a variety of applications, including in the speech-generating features of modern AAC technology. Researchers using ECoG and sEEG recordings have shown that it is possible to create speech BCIs that generate audible, intelligible speech from brain activity recorded as someone speaks, informed by parallel advances in TTS implementations.[40–42]

In one study, the researchers even synthesized speech from brain activity as the participant "mimed" or mouthed sentences (making articulatory movements as if they were saying the sentence but without vocalizing the sentence), which is an important step towards speech neuroprostheses where many future users will not be able to vocalize.[40] These studies laid important groundwork for future speech-neuroprosthetic research, proving that brain activity can be translated into speech acoustics using invasive neural recordings and modern AI techniques. As an alternative to directly decoding speech from brain activity, in practice a TTS synthesizer can instead be applied to decoded text to generate speech.

As a final point in this section, advances in non-invasive speech-decoding methods are briefly discussed. Although EEG typically exhibits lower signal resolution than invasive methods, researchers have been able to use EEG systems with modern AI approaches to decode speech,[23] with many studies focusing on decoding imagined speech (which involves the BCI user to imagine themselves saying something without actually saying it or moving their mouth) from brain activity.[24,25] Although not shown in Figure 3.1, another type of non-invasive neural-recording method is magnetoencephalography (MEG), which measures magnetic fields produced by the electrical activity in the brain. Researchers have shown that speech can be decoded from MEG recordings in real time.[22] However, MEG systems are currently not portable, and both EEG- and MEG-based speech BCIs have not approached the level of performance achieved with invasive techniques, although efforts to close this gap are still being actively pursued and non-invasive speech-BCI approaches are generally improving over time.

The First Speech Neuroprostheses

As methods for decoding speech from brain activity were refined and validated, new endeavors to design and create a speech neuroprosthesis with persons with severe paralysis and LiS became more justified. Before introducing the more recent speech-neuroprosthetic developments, the earliest effort towards a speech neuroprosthesis with a person with LiS involved a micro-electrode implanted in the SMC that enabled the participant to control a vowel synthesizer in real time,[43] and also facilitated offline decoding of linguistic sound units from brain activity.[44] Although performance was limited and the studies predated the breakthroughs in speech decoding described in the prior section, this effort represented an important early milestone in speech neuro-prosthetics by demonstrating that a person with LiS could control a BCI to generate speech-related outputs.

In 2019, researchers at the University of California, San Francisco, implanted an ECoG array over the SMC and neighboring brain areas of a man named Pancho, who suffered a brainstem stroke over 15 years prior to participation in the study that led to incomplete LiS (although he can still make some small movements, he is unable to articulate speech, walk, write, or type with his hands).[45] Pancho's brain activity was recorded as he attempted to say words from a 50-word vocabulary, and an AI model was created to learn the mapping between the ECoG signals and the words that he attempted to say. This model was used with a separately trained language model to enable Pancho to communicate in real time at 15 words per minute and 75% accuracy by attempting to say full sentences composed of words from the 50-word vocabulary.

This study proved for the first time that someone who had been unable to speak for years still retained functional representations of speech in their SMC that could drive a speech neuroprosthesis and enable communication in words and sentences. Subsequent work with Pancho demonstrated that a similar approach could be used to enable speech-based spelling for access to a larger vocabulary.[46] In the most recent work with Pancho, researchers created a bilingual speech neuroprosthesis that allowed Pancho to communicate in English and Spanish, with the ability to freely switch between the two languages between sentences.[10] This most recent study also provided evidence to support the longevity of ECoG-based speech neuroprostheses, with the data used in the study collected over 3.5 years after the implant of the ECoG array.

After the initial successes, the same research group implanted an upgraded ECoG array (with more recording sensors) over the SMC of a person named Ann, who also suffered a brainstem stroke over 15 years prior to participation in the study that caused incomplete LiS.[47] Ann's brain activity was recorded as she silently attempted to mouth (or "mime") sentences from a vocabulary of over 1,000 words. AI models were trained to learn the mapping between the recorded ECoG signals and linguistic, acoustic, and articulatory representations of the attempted sentences, enabling the decoding of text, speech sounds, and articulator movements (respectively) from brain activity. The researchers then showed that all three models could be used to decode sentences from Ann's brain activity in real time, output as text, synthesized speech, and animation of a facial avatar. The speech was synthesized in an artificial voice that was customized to sound like Ann (using a recording of her voice before her injury). The facial avatar was a 3-D digital character that had its mouth and face animated to correspond to decoded articulatory movements. This important milestone illustrated that text, speech, and other representations of expression can be restored to persons with LiS via a speech neuroprosthesis.

Encouraged by the initial proof-of-principle demonstrations with Pancho, other research institutions also began to explore the development of a speech neuroprosthesis. In one study, researchers demonstrated that a small set of keywords could be reliably synthesized from ECoG signals recorded as a man with impaired articulation due to amyotrophic lateral sclerosis (ALS) attempted to speak.[48] In another set of studies, MEAs were used to decode text from the brain activity of persons with impaired articulation due to ALS.[49,50] Performance was extremely favorable in one of these studies, enabling personal use of the speech neuroprosthesis for text and speech communication (through a TTS).[50] Questions around longevity and performance consistency across users of MEA-based speech neuroprostheses remain topics for ongoing work.

Speech Neuroprostheses as Assistive-Communication Devices

Findings and demonstrations from investigations of how speech is represented in the brain, efforts to decode speech from brain activity, initial implementations of speech neuroprostheses, and parallel advancements in AI techniques all support the growing feasibility of speech neuroprostheses as assistive-communication systems to improve expressivity of patients living with LiS. This concluding section focuses on how future speech neuroprostheses can serve as practical clinical solutions for patients, expanding their range of AAC options beyond traditional devices.

Multiple surveys have been conducted to assess what persons with LiS think and expect of communication BCIs.[51–54] In general, the survey respondents viewed BCI-based AACs favorably, although there are expectations of reliability and performance that need to be met before the risks and complexities of invasive BCIs can be warranted. Patients also reported that attempting to speak is a preferred method for controlling BCI-based AACs,[54] supporting speech neuroprostheses as useful AAC devices.

As technical studies push the boundaries of what is possible with speech neuroprostheses, the importance of addressing practical design aspects of the technology grows in parallel. Because speech decoding will not be perfect 100% of the time, speech neuroprostheses will need to include functionality to protect user agency, ensuring that decoded messages reflect the intent of the user.[55] Additionally, support for users to issue certain commands with extremely high reliability, which could be attempts to say certain phrases or make non-speech movements that are detectable from neural signals with near-perfect accuracy, should be considered for practical speech neuroprostheses.[55-57] Speech neuroprostheses should also be tightly integrated with the personal devices of patients to enable use of the technology for daily activities. Finally, the BCI devices themselves must be optimized for safety and long-term use, meaning that they should be fully implantable (so that the skin can fully heal after any implantation) and should not damage brain tissue.[10,55]

Although the potential of speech neuroprostheses is promising, any future decisions around receiving one of these devices must include careful considerations of the risks and limitations along with any anticipated benefits. One such limitation is that speech neuroprostheses generally rely on functional neuron populations in the SMC, meaning that the efficacy of these approaches in patients with SMC damage may be diminished. Although speech neuroprostheses have largely been demonstrated using recordings from left SMC (the human brain has two SMCs—one in the left hemisphere and one in the right), more research is needed to determine if recordings from the right SMC could be effective in patients with left-hemisphere damage.

Additionally, there have been early efforts to decode representations of speech and language outside of the SMC, offering another option for individuals with SMC damage.[58,59] However, cortical neurodegeneration, which occurs in diseases like ALS and involves the degradation of neural populations in the cortex, may hinder decoding performance over time.[60] It may be possible to maximize the efficacy of a speech neuroprosthesis by beginning to use it before significant neurodegeneration, which should improve training of the speech-decoding models via higher fidelity neural signals, but this could involve surgical intervention before full loss of communication capabilities, and thus would need to be carefully considered and supported by further research.

Another limitation of current speech neuroprostheses is that they might not be effective for patients with LiS that also have significant cognitive deficits, as the user must be capable of comprehending language and attempting to speak for the approach to work. Finally, the best-performing speech neuroprostheses all require invasive surgery, which is a serious medical procedure that carries risks. In general, speech neuroprostheses may not be suitable for every person with LiS, and future users should consult with their clinical teams to determine which types of AACs are most appropriate given their specific conditions and needs (Figure 3.2).

Despite current limitations, the progress made in speech-neuroprosthetic research in the past decade is remarkable and encouraging. Enabled by advances in speech neuroscience, BCI hardware development, and related AI fields, research institutions and companies across the globe are pursuing the development of speech neuroprostheses to help patients with LiS communicate. Although traditional AAC devices will likely continue to be an

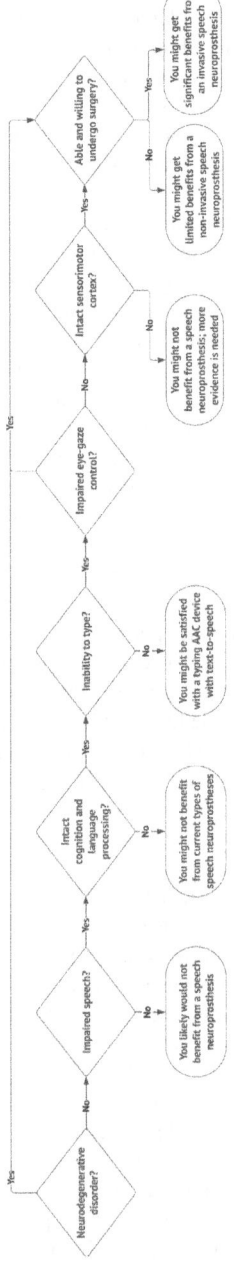

Figure 3.2 Flowchart for speech-neuroprosthesis suitability. Decision nodes are in diamonds and endpoints are in ovals. For individuals who need AAC technology but are not recommended to get a BCI, traditional AAC technology may be more suitable. Note that impaired eye-gaze control might warrant the consideration of a BCI despite a damaged SMC due to limitations in the number of other viable options for that patient. Note that these suitability depictions are not medical recommendations, and the suitability of speech neuroprostheses for any given person should be discussed with clinical teams once speech neuroprostheses are available for purchase.

important part of the ecosystem for years to come, speech neuroprostheses are poised to transform the way that AAC technology can restore expressivity to patients.

As progress continues to be made toward clinically viable solutions, it is important to acknowledge the sacrifices made by those who volunteer to participate in the studies that drive this progress. People like Pancho and Ann undergo surgery to receive investigational BCIs and dedicate significant portions of their time and energy, sometimes for 5+ years, in hopes of accelerating the science and eventually improving the lives of people they have never met.[61] Shared by researchers, engineers, clinicians, and patients around the world, this hope for improved communication for patients with LiS gets closer to reality each day, driven by growth and innovation toward the development of a clinically viable speech neuroprosthesis and the BCI pioneers who selflessly enable this progress.

Editor's note: Please see chapter 7 for details of Ann Johnson's experience of BCIs with Dr. David Moses and the team at the Chang Lab at UCSF.

For further information and a more thorough, technical explanation about speech neuroprostheses, this is a helpful review: https://www.nature.com/articles/s41583-024-00819-9.

References

1. Rousseau MC, Baumstarck K, Alessandrini M, Blandin V, Billette de Villemeur T, Auquier P. Quality of life in patients with locked-in syndrome: evolution over a 6-year period. Orphanet J Rare Dis. 2015;10:88. doi:10.1186/s13023-015-0304-z

2. Felgoise SH, Zaccheo V, Duff J, Simmons Z. Verbal communication impacts quality of life in patients with amyotrophic lateral sclerosis. Amyotroph Lateral Scler Front Degener. 2016;17(3-4):179–183. doi:10.3109/21678421.2015.1125499

3. Martin Pistorius, How my mind came back to life - and no one knew. TED Conf. Published online 2015. https://www.ted.com/talks/martin_pistorius_how_my_mind_came_back_to_life_and_no_one_knew?subtitle=en

4. Beukelman DR, Fager S, Ball L, Dietz A. AAC for adults with acquired neurological conditions: a review. Augment Altern Commun. 2007;23(3):230–242. doi:10.1080/07434610701553668

5. Linse K, Aust E, Joos M, Hermann A, Oliver DJ. Communication matters—pitfalls and promise of hightech communication devices in palliative care of severely physically disabled patients with amyotrophic lateral sclerosis. Front Neurol. 2018;9(July):1–18. doi:10.3389/fneur.2018.00603

6. Johnson JM, Inglebret E, Jones C, Ray J. Perspectives of speech language pathologists regarding success versus abandonment of AAC. Augment Altern Commun. 2006;22(2):85–99. doi:10.1080/07434610500483588

7. Brumberg JS, Pitt KM, Mantie-Kozlowski A, Burnison JD. Brain-computer interfaces for augmentative and alternative communication: a tutorial. Am J Speech Lang Pathol. 2018;27(1):1–12. doi:10.1044/2017_AJSLP-16-0244

8. Chaudhary U, Birbaumer N, Ramos-Murguialday A. Brain-computer interfaces for communication and rehabilitation. Nat Rev Neurol. 2016;12(9):513–525. doi:10.1038/nrneurol.2016.113

9. Chang EF, Anumanchipalli GK. Toward a speech neuroprosthesis. JAMA. 2019;323(5):413. doi:10.1001/jama.2019.19813

10. Silva AB, Littlejohn KT, Liu JR, Moses DA, Chang EF. The speech neuroprosthesis. Nat Rev Neurosci. 2024;25(7):473–492. doi:10.1038/s41583-024-00819-9

11. Moses DA, Chang EF, Wilson BS, et al. Toward a direct-speech neuroprosthesis: decoding speech from sensorimotor cortex using artificial intelligence. In: Harnessing the power of artificial intelligence in otolaryngology and the communication sciences. Vol 23. Journal of the Association for Research in Otolaryngology; 2022:322–327.

12. Bouchard KE, Mesgarani N, Johnson K, Chang EF. Functional organization of human sensorimotor cortex for speech articulation. Nature. 2013;495(7441):327–332. doi:10.1038/nature11911

13. Carey D, Krishnan S, Callaghan MF, Sereno MI, Dick F. Functional and quantitative MRI mapping of somatomotor representations of human supralaryngeal vocal tract. Cereb Cortex. 2017;27(1):265–278. doi:10.1093/cercor/bhw393

14. Penfield W, Boldrey E. Somatic motor and sensory representation in the cerebral cortex of man as studied by electrical stimulation. Brain. 1937;60(4):389–443.

15. Cushing H. A note upon the faradic stimulation of the postcentral gyrus in conscious patients. Brain. 1909;32(1):44–53.

16. Penfield W, Rasmussen T. The cerebral cortex of man; a clinical study of localization of function. Macmillan, 1950.

17. Chakrabarti S, Sandberg HM, Brumberg JS, Krusienski DJ. Progress in speech decoding from the electrocorticogram. Biomed Eng Lett. 2015;5(1):10–21. doi:10.1007/s13534-015-0175-1

18. Lotte F, Brumberg JS, Brunner P, et al. Electrocorticographic representations of segmental features in continuous speech. Front Hum Neurosci. 2015;09(February):1–13. doi:10.3389/fnhum.2015.00097

19. Dichter BK, Breshears JD, Leonard MK, Chang EF. The control of vocal pitch in human laryngeal motor cortex. Cell. 2018;174(1):1–11. doi:10.1016/j.cell.2018.05.016

20. Conant DF, Bouchard KE, Leonard MK, Chang EF. Human sensorimotor cortex control of directly-measured vocal tract movements during vowel production. J Neurosci. 2018;38(12):2955–2956. doi:10.1523/JNEUROSCI.2382-17.2018

21. Akcakaya M, Peters B, Moghadamfalahi M, et al. Noninvasive brain–computer interfaces for augmentative and alternative communication. IEEE Rev Biomed Eng. 2014;7:31–49. doi:10.1109/RBME.2013.2295097

22. Dash D, Ferrari P, Wang J. Decoding imagined and spoken phrases from non-invasive neural (MEG) signals. Front Neurosci. 2020;14:290. doi:10.3389/fnins.2020.00290

23. Shah U, Alzubaidi M, Mohsen F, Abd-Alrazaq A, Alam T, Househ M. The role of artificial intelligence in decoding speech from EEG signals: a scoping review. Sensors. 2022;22(18):6975. doi:10.3390/s22186975

24. Lopez-Bernal D, Balderas D, Ponce P, Molina A. A state-of-the-art review of EEG-based imagined speech decoding. Front Hum Neurosci. 2022;16:867281. doi:10.3389/fnhum.2022.867281

25. Panachakel JT, Ramakrishnan AG. Decoding covert speech from EEG-a comprehensive review. Front Neurosci. 2021;15:642251. doi:10.3389/fnins.2021. 642251

26. Gold B, Morgan N, Ellis D. Speech and audio signal processing: processing and perception of speech and music. 2nd ed. John Wiley & Sons, Inc.; 2011. https:// books.google.com/books?id=p0mNAF8gMmUC

27. Graves A, Mohamed A rahman, Hinton G. Speech recognition with deep recurrent neural networks. In: International conference on acoustics, speech, and signal processing.; 2013:6645–6649. doi:10.1109/ICASSP.2013.6638947

28. Wang D, Wang X, Lv S. An overview of end-to-end automatic speech recognition. Symmetry. 2019;11(8):1018. doi:10.3390/sym11081018

29. Herff C, Schultz T. Automatic speech recognition from neural signals: a focused review. Front Neurosci. 2016;10. doi:10.3389/fnins.2016.00429

30. Chen SF, Goodman J. An empirical study of smoothing techniques for language modeling. Comput Speech Lang. 1999;13(4):359–393. doi:10.1006/csla.1999.0128

31. Herff C, Heger D, de Pesters A, et al. Brain-to-text: decoding spoken phrases from phone representations in the brain. Front Neurosci. 2015;9(June):1–11. doi:10.3389/fnins.2015.00217

32. Moses DA, Leonard MK, Makin JG, Chang EF. Real-time decoding of question-and-answer speech dialogue using human cortical activity. Nat Commun. 2019;10(1):3096. doi:10.1038/s41467-019-10994-4

33. Sun P, Anumanchipalli GK, Chang EF. Brain2Char: a deep architecture for decoding text from brain recordings. J Neural Eng. 2020;17(6):066015. doi:10.1088/ 1741-2552/abc742

34. Makin JG, Moses DA, Chang EF. Machine translation of cortical activity to text with an encoder–decoder framework. Nat Neurosci. 2020;23(4):575–582. doi:10.1038/s41593-020-0608-8

35. Murray IR, Arnott JL. Toward the simulation of emotion in synthetic speech: A review of the literature on human vocal emotion. J Acoust Soc Am. 1993;93(2): 1097–1108. doi:10.1121/1.405558

36. Dutoit T. An introduction to text-to-speech synthesis. Vol 3. Springer Science & Business Media; 1997.

37. Oord A van den, Dieleman S, Zen H, et al. WaveNet: a generative model for raw audio. ArXiv160903499 Cs. September 19, 2016. http://arxiv.org/abs/1609.03499

38. Ning Y, He S, Wu Z, Xing C, Zhang LJ. A review of deep learning based speech synthesis. Appl Sci. 2019;9(19):4050. doi:10.3390/app9194050

39. Ling ZH, Richmond K, Yamagishi J, Wang RH. Integrating articulatory features into HMM-based parametric speech synthesis. IEEE Trans Audio Speech Lang Process. 2009;17(6):1171–1185. doi:10.1109/TASL.2009.2014796

40. Anumanchipalli GK, Chartier J, Chang EF. Speech synthesis from neural decoding of spoken sentences. Nature. 2019;568(7753):493–498. doi:10.1038/s41586-019-1119-1

41. Angrick M, Herff C, Mugler E, et al. Speech synthesis from ECoG using densely connected 3D convolutional neural networks. J Neural Eng. 2019;16(3):036019. doi:10.1088/1741-2552/ab0c59

42. Angrick M, Ottenhoff MC, Diener L, et al. Real-time synthesis of imagined speech processes from minimally invasive recordings of neural activity. Commun Biol. 2021;4(1):1055. doi:10.1038/s42003-021-02578-0

43. Guenther FH, Brumberg JS, Wright EJ, et al. A wireless brain-machine interface for real-time speech synthesis. Ben-Jacob E, ed. PLOS ONE. 2009;4(12):e8218. doi:10.1371/journal.pone.0008218

44. Brumberg JS, Wright EJ, Andreasen DS, Guenther FH, Kennedy PR. Classification of intended phoneme production from chronic intracortical microelectrode recordings in speech-motor cortex. Front Neurosci. May 12, 2011. doi:10.3389/fnins.2011.00065

45. Moses DA, Metzger SL, Liu JR, et al. Neuroprosthesis for decoding speech in a paralyzed person with anarthria. N Engl J Med. 2021;385(3):217–227. doi:10.1056/NEJMoa2027540

46. Metzger SL, Liu JR, Moses DA, et al. Generalizable spelling using a speech neuroprosthesis in an individual with severe limb and vocal paralysis. Nat Commun. 2022;13(1):6510. doi:10.1038/s41467-022-33611-3

47. Metzger SL, Littlejohn KT, Silva AB, et al. A high-performance neuroprosthesis for speech decoding and avatar control. Nature. August 23, 2023. doi:10.1038/s41586-023-06443-4

48. Angrick M, Luo S, Rabbani Q, et al. Online speech synthesis using a chronically implanted brain-computer interface in an individual with ALS. Sci Rep. 2024;14(1):9617. doi:10.1038/s41598-024-60277-2

49. Willett FR, Kunz EM, Fan C, et al. A high-performance speech neuroprosthesis. Nature. 2023;620(7976):1031–1036. doi:10.1038/s41586-023-06377-x

50. Card NS, Wairagkar M, Iacobacci C, et al. An accurate and rapidly calibrating speech neuroprosthesis. N Engl J Med. 2024;391(7):609–618. doi:10.1056/NEJMoa2314132

51. Huggins JE, Wren PA, Gruis KL. What would brain-computer interface users want? Opinions and priorities of potential users with amyotrophic lateral sclerosis. Amyotroph Lateral Scler. 2011;12(5):318–324. doi:10.3109/17482968.2011.572978

52. Lahr J, Schwartz C, Heimbach B, Aertsen A, Rickert J, Ball T. Invasive brain-machine interfaces: a survey of paralyzed patients' attitudes, knowledge and methods of information retrieval. J Neural Eng. 2015;12(4). doi:10.1088/1741-2560/12/4/043001

53. Kageyama Y, He X, Shimokawa T, et al. Nationwide survey of 780 Japanese patients with amyotrophic lateral sclerosis: their status and expectations from brain-machine interfaces. J Neurol. 2020;267(10):2932–2940. doi:10.1007/s00415-020-09903-3

54. Branco MP, Pels EGM, Sars RH, et al. Brain-computer interfaces for communication: preferences of individuals with locked-in syndrome. Neurorehabil Neural Repair. 2021;35(3):267–279. doi:10.1177/1545968321989331

55. Sankaran N, Moses D, Chiong W, Chang EF. Recommendations for promoting user agency in the design of speech neuroprostheses. Front Hum Neurosci. 2023;17:1298129. doi:10.3389/fnhum.2023.1298129

56. Hurtig RR, Alper RM, Bryant KNT, Davidson KR, Bilskemper C. Improving patient safety and patient–provider communication. perspect ASHA spec interest groups. 2019;4(5):1017–1027. doi:10.1044/2019_PERS-SIG12-2019-0021

57. Chandler JA, Van Der Loos KI, Boehnke S, Beaudry JS, Buchman DZ, Illes J. Brain computer interfaces and communication disabilities: ethical, legal, and social aspects of decoding speech from the brain. Front Hum Neurosci. 2022;16:841035. doi:10.3389/fnhum.2022.841035

58. Tang J, LeBel A, Jain S, Huth AG. Semantic reconstruction of continuous language from non-invasive brain recordings. Nat Neurosci. 2023;26(5):858–866. doi:10.1038/s41593-023-01304-9

59. Wandelt SK, Bjånes DA, Pejsa K, Lee B, Liu C, Andersen RA. Representation of internal speech by single neurons in human supramarginal gyrus. Nat Hum Behav. 2024;8(6):1136–1149. doi:10.1038/s41562-024-01867-y

60. Vansteensel MJ, Leinders S, Branco MP, et al. Longevity of a brain-computer interface for amyotrophic lateral sclerosis. N Engl J Med. 2024;391(7):619–626. doi:10.1056/NEJMoa2314598

61. Patrick-Krueger KM, Burkhart I, Contreras-Vidal JL. The state of clinical trials of implantable brain–computer interfaces. Nat Rev Bioeng. September 20, 2024. doi:10.1038/s44222-024-00239-5

4 "It Doesn't Bend That Way"

Duncan R. Campling

Birthed and educated in London, England. At 24, I chose to emigrate to America for professional reasons. 1996 was the exact year, and I eventually lived in the Upper East Side of Manhattan, and worked in the iconic Empire State Building. NYC was constantly evolving, and I was excited to be working at the intersection of technology and Wall Street finance. It was an incredible and pivotal time. Cell phones were busy shrinking, and Manhattan was rightly at the center of the universe.

By 2018, the year of my two strokes, I had become a lead technical recruiter for Amazon Corporate in Seattle, and separately Etsy's global HQ in Brooklyn. In essence, I consulted with software development managers or directors to buildout their teams of programmers and software designers. For recreation, I enjoyed lounging poolside, camping and playing electric guitar until my house literally shook. However my American dream would soon take a dramatic turn…

One sunny 2018 March morning at my home in suburban Philadelphia, I called my manager in Brooklyn, New York, informing him that I urgently needed to take a power-nap, as I had an earth-shattering headache. Phoning my manager was one of the niceties of working from home. As I slowly drifted off, I tried slightly adjusting my position, but I awoke suddenly. To my horror, I realized I was paralyzed head-to-toe, and was only able to blink!

Eventually Ed, my kitchen contractor found me. He wanted to show me his progress, but soon realized I was in a medical crisis, and promptly alerted my then wife, who was downstairs. She was advised by the emergency services to proceed with CPR, however I remained trapped within. Astonishingly, I had a brief out of body experience. From my master bedroom ceiling, I somehow viewed my wife frantically give me chest compressions. Was I already dreaming?

The ambulance arrived, and my lifeless body was swiftly transferred from the warm, comforting embrace of my bed, to an emergency stretcher. The first responders wrongly assumed I must have overdosed on hard drugs. At 47, they figured I was too young to have something like a stroke. That's why I never received clot busting TPA drugs for my first stroke. During the

DOI: 10.4324/9781003464181-4

ambulance ride one of the first responders actually said to his colleague while looking at my face, "can I call it?" After immediately ascertaining he was referring to my time of death, I wanted to loudly exclaim, "CAN'T YOU TELL I'M STILL ALIVE?!" However the mind/muscle connections from my brain to my mouth had apparently been severed. No words came out.

Before long, I was skilfully lowered into a nearby hospital ICU bed. A small team of medics gathered around, and an overwhelming collection of tubes and wires were attached to me. Like a dog on a leash, I was tethered.

A young affable male nurse told me he had a Transient Ischemic Attack (TIA, aka mini-stroke) in his late teens, and personally did all his own physical rehab. Previously, I thought rehab was for alcoholics and drug users, battling addiction. I now know differently.

My brother, who lived not that far from me, explained to my motionless frame that he had helped his friend in England recover from stroke. This gave me some much needed hope. He quickly became friends with one of the nursing aides, which was fortunate because I wanted nursing staff to like me, so they'd give me their best medical care. Even leaving me slightly twisted had painful consequences. I had suddenly become at everyone's mercy.

One of my nursing aides was a massive Jamaican woman, towering high above me. My brother talked with her about Jamaican curry. However all I could think about was that she was a colossal ball of a woman. So tall and round, she had visible difficulty walking. If she put one foot wrong she had the potential to crush me. Why was I here? By now I was told I had had a stroke. But strokes were for much older, or seriously unfit people, weren't they? Evidently not.

My instinctive swallow was so weak, a feeding tube had to be surgically implanted in my stomach. Basically a liquid food bag was attached to a pump, and then suspended from a pole. Nothing by mouth for now. Nursing staff also had to wrap me in blankets in my wheelchair because I was unable to regulate my own body temperature. A function I had previously taken for granted, but it was now an unattainable luxury. The following week, I had a swallow study scheduled with a fun & cute speech therapist to see if I could now take any food by mouth.

Unfortunately our session was cut short, as I had some traumatic neurological event. A bulletin was issued over the hospital speakers. Immediately 20 panicked doctors and neurologists arrived, taking turns to shake their heads and comforting me like someone had just died. I later learned the neurological event was a second ischemic, brain stem stroke. It was a painless experience, and strangely there was almost a hidden peace about it. The first stroke seemed relatively manageable, but the second sent me deep under. However I wrongly assumed this was a very temporary situation, and everything would probably blow over in two weeks, three tops.

Like vultures, doctors circled above me, and they all wanted to shine their flashlights in my eyes and wiggle my toes. Apparently, my blood clot had somehow moved from the left side to the right side of my brain. I'm no medic, but I guess that explains why both sides of my body were paralyzed (and now significantly weakened). Unfortunately I was informed that I was not a viable candidate for a craniotomy because the exact area of my brain stem was too intricate, and thus inoperable. Additionally, there was no active cure. My medications were just a cocktail of painkillers, anticoagulants, antidepressants and sleeping pills. So there was nothing to make me whole again. Current treatment for LiS is just to make sufferers feel more comfortable. A doctor explained to my wife in private that my physical recovery had plateaued, and if I showed any further improvements they would be very minor. The prognosis seemed dire, and was so extreme it felt like a giant conspiracy against me.

Ten days after my strokes, my divorced parents and stepmother visited from England. My father advised me, "you'll have to think your way out of this one." Probably because my brain needed to build alternative pathways (neuroplasticity). My mother and father flew back separately after a few days. Thankfully my stepmother was able to stay for a couple more months.

When thinking about my boys, who must have been very concerned, I often thought, "I'm going through this so you don't have to." If only that was true. I was later told by a great neurologist who oversaw months of tests, that my two strokes were probably not genetic, but cryptogenic, which is just a fancy medical term for, "we still have no idea of the cause."

Standing at 6'3", almost 6'4", I've always been proud to be quite tall. However in US hospitals, I was commonly referred by nursing staff to as, "Way too long." For some reason nearly all equipment is built for people up to 6 foot. Nursing aides often treat me like I'm 7'3". My height had become an inconvenience for everyone involved, even me.

Week two, a small neurology team formally diagnosed me with LiS. Although, they previously acknowledged that I was fully aware and "in there". Binary questions were answered with one blink for "yes" and two blinks for "no". However I would blink once for "yes", but shortly afterwards I would often accidentally blink once again. This was interpreted as a "no", or deemed inconclusive.

I titled my chapter, "It Doesn't Bend That Way" because while being washed and dressed, my nursing aides would sometimes attempt to manipulate my limbs like a pretzel. Thankfully, they were unsuccessful, but I was unable to complain or redirect. The objective of my chapter is to inform similar folks they're not alone.

One of my aides defined the phrase, "Charlie Horse" to her colleague, while washing me. I was intrigued because I had not heard it before, but I didn't know just how relatable the term would become. A Charlie Horse apparently refers to an itch you just can't reach to scratch. The phrase had suddenly become highly relatable.

Now I could nod and shake my head, which made answering binary questions much easier. Consequently I was able to spell out words using a laser pointer taped to a baseball cap. My brother had the laser pointer project on a large alphabet board. Unsurprisingly, my first word was, "T R A N S F E R" because I wanted to expedite this medical experience.

I've always believed, you are what you do, and I was proud of my professional achievements thus far. Nevertheless to most people my previous self was totally irrelevant to them, and everything was all about my new incarnation, Duncan 2.0. I would later mourn the loss of Duncan 1.0. Inadvertently I had let stroke define me, but I wasn't defeated just yet. A therapist showed me that my hospital bed moved into the shape of a chair. We sat on the edge together. I didn't know it then, but this was the first step of my physical rehabilitation journey. My mental and emotional rehabilitation would start six years later.

After requesting a transfer out of the ICU, I was eventually whisked off by ambulance to an intensive, acute rehabilitation facility. No siren was necessary this time though. In the grounds of my new facility lay a pond complete with schools of carp, a few snapping turtles and a resident heron. There was even a basketball hoop, which I imagine served as a recovery incentive. Had I transferred to some medical nirvana?

My back and legs felt like they were nailed to my wheelchair, but my speech therapist provided me with an eye-gaze equipped iPad to allow me to communicate more effectively. Two small cameras at the base of the device looked at my pupils, to see where I was staring on a keyboard, as I had no use of my hands yet. The only problem was the cameras weren't accurately calibrated. I had to stare at 'M' to type a 'N', which obviously proved problematic. The technology had the beginnings of being awesome, but the execution was underwhelming back then. Hopefully it has improved since my unsuccessful attempts in 2018.

Conversely, the gym at the acute rehab was perfectly tailored and well conceived. Like some tortured marionette, their walking robot involved me being suspended by a harness over a slow moving treadmill. I also wore an exoskeleton strapped to me, that was cleverly designed to correct my gait. Initially the contraption did most of the walking for me, but the physical therapists operating it decreased the assistance it offered, by lowering the weight support from the harness. Funnily, the contraption closely resembled the main character from the movie, RoboCop.

Hooray, I could finally move my right arm and fingers. It thankfully meant I no longer was forced to use the tedious eye-gaze technology to communicate as I was now capable of pressing the keyboard on a large iPad. One finger on one hand is how I type to this day. As you can imagine, I'm a habitual user of predictive text to finish my "swords":) Seriously, after a few months I was eternally grateful to be on a path to recovery, as many LiS people literally suffer without making significant gains for multiple decades!

My acute facility had an intensive six hour a day therapy regimen, designed to accelerate physical and speech recover. I pushed myself hard, and diligently did my "homework" as recovery from this living nightmare had rapidly become my sole mission. Most stroke survivors have already lived their lives. At 47 I urgently needed to get back to my young family, but Duncan 1.0 was fading and almost a distant memory. Unlike many older stroke survivors, I had more parenting and living to do. Like switching a light on and off, I innocently assumed stroke recovery would be a sudden event, but my path remains more gradual and non-linear. The ancient proverb of Lao Tsu, "the journey of a thousand miles begins with one step," never seemed more relevant.

One fellow patient was a 19 year old young man. He was badly hurt in a motorcycle accident, and remained in a coma. Amazingly with electrodes strategically attached to various muscle groups, he was able to slightly move his limbs. To my eternal frustration, he actually made faster progress than me! However we were both starting from the same place; zero. I keep telling myself his youth must have given him a slight edge on me.

In speech therapy I spelled out on an alphabet board, "D I D I D I E?" This was my only explanation for my current predicament. However it was later relayed to me that in fact I did not die, but I did flatline in the ambulance. That probably explained why the first responders declared my time of death.

My lead physical therapist had two assistants. Collectively, their good humor helped the time pass as I busily worked out in the gym. During therapy they gave me simple card games to play, which kept me sufficiently distracted, while I eagerly awaited their next instruction. An occupational therapist also had me test drive an electric powered wheelchair. The head nurse in my section jokingly asked me to give her a ride to the local convenience store, but the powered wheelchair was limited to a maximum speed of 0.5 mph.

As you can imagine "emotional incontinence" is when you can't control your emotions. I would alarmingly transition from crying to laughing, with no midway point. Medically it's called Pseudobulbar Affect, or PBA for short. The condition has definitely lessened with time, but I still have some tendencies. Thinking of my boys often triggers my PBA, but laughing at funerals is the classic textbook example. In addition, I had become extremely irritable, and would fly off the handle over very minor issues. My anger would go from 0 to 100 mph in an instant. People didn't know how to react, as I apparently have zero filter left.

My acute rehabilitation time had come to an abrupt end, and I was informed three hours before that I was to be shipped off to a nursing home for old people. This was particularly soul crushing because I knew it was a long-term solution. So I spent my final hours begging staff on my alphabet board to "S A V E M E." My once beloved acute rehab facility had seemingly given up and betrayed me. In reality there was little they could do for me, and new patients needed the bed.

At the new nursing home, I officially became a gym rat, exercising five or six days a week. LiS recovery takes no vacations or public holidays. The only notable difference between weekends and weekdays, is weekends involve less therapy.

Being on public assistance I had to share a bedroom and bathroom with another resident. When I moved into my first nursing home my roommate was starving himself to death. A week later, he would be successful. His friend stopped by a few days later, to pick up his personals. My freshly deceased roommate was my closest brush with mortality. A replacement was promptly assigned to occupy his bed. My new roommate's illness was completely invisible. I overheard him tell a psychologist he regularly heard voices in his head. Thankfully, the voices didn't tell him to murder his defenceless roommate in his sleep. His sister lived in Colorado, and after two months, he thankfully went to live with her.

Enter Joe. Joe was a ninety-something "trouble maker", and constantly gave the nursing staff a difficult time with his endless rants and harmless fist fights. Unlike me, he could talk up a storm. His rants were comedy gold, but intended seriously. Apparently he was well built when he arrived at the nursing home, but time and lack of use had a badly atrophied his frame. Like many residents, he refused ALL exercise, even therapy. However Joe could stand up by himself and walk a bit, but shook like a leaf doing so. He made me feel extremely vulnerable during his nightly attempts because I knew I would be unable to fend him off if he fell on me. Joe often struggled with reality too, which only highlighted my anxiety.

Drug addicts often refer to "hitting rock bottom." I'm no drug addict, but hitting rock bottom for me was probably when I contracted pneumonia and a gallbladder infection, which quickly led to sepsis. After surgical recovery at hospital, I switched to a better and cleaner nursing home.

Two years post stroke, my developing core muscles allowed me to lean forward in my wheelchair. This enabled me to brush my teeth over a sink. Leaning forward also allowed me access to the drawers in my cabinets. I found the drawers were half full of trash, like the ripped wrapping paper from a birthday present. Why would anyone possibly want to keep that junk?

Sleeping was still a major issue. For the first two years, I was often sleepless for 72 hours straight! Most of the issue was neurological, but the television across the hallway was so loud, and left on 24/7 because the owner was hard of hearing, and he liked it permanently on. His TV was often on for months, even years. Until one day he passed from old age. I tried to play chess with my neighbor's 12 year old son. Predictably, due to extreme sleep deprivation, I played like a rookie. Losing, understandably damaged my already weak ego.

Neurofatigue is real, and feels very different to being just dog tired. You feel like an insomniac zombie, walking through molasses. For me, intense fatigue can come on in 30 seconds. I have to immediately stop what I'm doing and shutdown. Extreme energy loss during the day forced me to become an expert in time management, allowing for appropriate rest periods between activities. I often meditate to accelerate rest during the day. When I want to sleep I normally have trouble, so I resort to sleeping pills.

Year three post strokes, I started walking with a walker, and help from multiple physical therapists. My first attempt was just eight feet, but I was ecstatic just to be steppin' again.

At that time too, I saw many professional athletes were new vegans. Thankfully I could eat regular food one year after the stroke. For the apparent physical benefits of veganism, I became one too, but after two months I missed cheese too much, and became vegetarian instead. That lasted for a further 10 months, before becoming a pescatarian, and eventually a card carrying carnivore again.

I'm not expecting restaurant quality from my nursing home, but any positive nutrients from my vegetables had already been stewed out, and thrown away with the water.

While I could eat regular food, regular water was another story, as it moves around in the throat too quickly, and fluid can enter the lungs, causing pneumonia. After many swallow studies over five long years, I was formally graduated to thin liquids (regular water). I could now eat and drink absolutely anything! This was a mammoth goal accomplished. Whoever counted me out after 12 months, obviously can't count.

One day I attended a trivia session hosted by someone from the Recreation Department. They were reading questions from the popular game, Trivial Pursuit. I enjoyed it so much I attended again the next day too. However there was a completely different crowd, even the person hosting. I was surprised she read the exact same questions from the previous day. I didn't say anything because I thought I can have fun with this. Remembering 95% of the correct answers, I was answering before the questions were even finished. Everyone in the room was amazed and several jaws dropped. They thought I could see the answers on the card, or was looking at mirrors. However their defense measures were futile, and no one could work out how I was doing it. I left for lunch, and forgot to tell them how I knew all the correct answers. Maybe they're still talking about it now.

For something else positive to do, I rekindled a deep interest in gardening. In some ways gardening also recreated the nurturing scenario of being a parent. A friendly staff member asked the general manager if I could grow something outside in the nursing home garden. Surprisingly she agreed, and for the first year I grew super hot Thai chili peppers and cherry tomatoes. With watering, pruning, harvesting and fall clean-up, the experience also served as excellent occupational therapy for fine motor skills. Raising and nurturing something from seed was extremely satisfying too.

Not that I've tried actual driving post stroke, my auto driving license was downgraded to just a basic ID. The loss was emblematic of losing my hard fought freedom decades ago. Post strokes I used a realistic driving simulator once, but unfortunately my average reaction time to emergency stops was double the suggested minimum for real driving. Although I already knew I was unsafe to drive because in the first 15 minutes of the simulation, I flipped the car twice by mounting the curb at speed. I was mildly annoyed, but grateful it wasn't real life.

From thousands of oral motor exercises, my breath control had progressed so I could achieve adequate speech volume. Consequently I became able to properly blow my nose again. For the first time in almost six years, my nasal passages were completely cleared. It felt so liberating not to be a mouth breather anymore. Finally some relief and welcome civilization.

Incidentally I was the youngest patient in my nursing home by several years. Many of the other residents will never be able to bounce back because they had dementia, Alzheimer's, Parkinson's, or were just plain old. Staff who don't know me, often bundle me in with these poor folks, and reject any progress I have managed to make thus far. They become alarmed and disturbed when I rightfully give them the middle finger.

Apparently 80% of stroke survivors get divorced before or after their stroke. Compared with 50% of "regular people". I officially became another statistic in 2023. Duncan 2.0 then had to transition to Duncan 3.0, the post divorce version of me. Over 19 years of marriage, we had eventually drifted apart. Understandably, I miss living with my two young boys very much. They both know I'm their dad, but we've lived separately for way too long. I mostly miss sleeping under the same roof as them, and being more present in their lives.

When walking, my height adds to my fear of falling. At 6'3" I have slightly further to fall than average, but I also have a higher center of gravity to keep balanced. I had eight stitches on my eyebrow, the only time I fell, and that was from a seated position.

In my experience, medical gaslighting is alive and well in US nursing homes. I am regularly treated like a six year old, or a "confused" older person. I know I'm neither, but it's super-frustrating because my voice is less intelligible the more upset I become. Furthermore, the offending gaslighters often leave before understanding what I was trying to say.

Any idiosyncrasy is written off by nursing aides as sheer lunacy. To add insult to injury, I scored 30 out of 30 on a cognition test in 2023. The doctor who tested me, openly admitted he'd probably score less. One of my roommates rarely responded to his name (or anything). Even though difficult to watch for his family, it must have been blissful to be that oblivious and unaware.

While listening to my favorite podcast, I realized I have photosensitivity post strokes. I prefer to do most activities without main lights on, especially fluorescent lights, which are everywhere in nursing homes. I try to rely on natural light from windows, anything else often seems overwhelming.

Stroke has taught me patience. Duncan 1.0 wanted everything on a plate, immediately. Whereas these days, I'm happy taking my time because I know I can out wait anyone. Patience has become my new superpower.

Everyone else's lives move forward without me. New movies are filmed, and therapists accept new job offers etc. Conversely my life remains static. Did the clocks go forward a few years, leaving me behind? Life is still a constant struggle, but I am now capable of walking over 200 ft with a walker and physical therapist in tow. Additionally, I'm able to stand up without any assistance. Lastly according to my speech therapist, I'm about 85% intelligible. These were weighty wins, and all accomplished through relentless exercise. In my experience, there are no magic pills or shortcuts to rapid stroke recovery.

Brain health is equally as important as physical fitness. For me, I like to keep my brain busy with multiple online word games. They're also relaxing, satisfying and healthier than watching TV. I'm no saint, but there's a reason people call TV the "idiot box". Thinking aids the recovery process as you're constantly searching for new scenarios, building new connections and keeping the mind active and well oiled.

Staff who don't know me, often assume I was born in Pennsylvania, and I must be over 80 because I live in a nursing home. Some even talk in a slow, loud voice because they wrongly assume I'm mentally challenged, or possibly deaf. My very identity is constantly under threat, so I created an informative one page bio for just outside my room.

With time, what I thought were enduring, lifelong friendships, often fade to black. I also chose to end all toxic ties, although, a few strong friendships survived the cull.

Like switching a light on and off, I assumed I would suddenly be 'fixed'. I later discovered stroke recovery is gradual, an ongoing process, built from many small wins and milestones. I'm often told each win needs to be celebrated, regardless how incremental. Personally, I choose to celebrate with an inspiring Instagram post. Fellow stroke survivors and LiS folk often comment, offering their love and support. Consequently, they give me the fire to push on even harder.

My thoughts on adaptive technologies aimed at disabled people are, "they're good for certain people", and were a useful transition for me, but not good if introduced as a permanent solution to a problem because they imply I won't progress further. I should add that my theory does not apply to amputees, or anyone that needs a permanent solution.

Most people still try unnecessarily to assist me the second I show any effort, but all I want is to be left alone, and to be as independent as possible. So I normally wait for absolutely everyone to leave the room, before attempting anything. Physically, my ultimate goal is not to regain everything I lost, but to eventually live completely independently. I know it's a lofty goal, but larger feats seemed unachievable at first.

Fast forward to present day, I'm more accepting of Duncan 3.0 (post strokes & divorce). For me recovery is a slow, perpetual process. I think Desmond Tutu said it best, "there is only one way to eat an elephant: one bite a time."

A minority of stroke survivors are never able to return to work. Sadly, I'm currently one of them, and as a result, I'm unable to provide for my kids the way I once did. For example: my firstborn son was planning to celebrate his thirteenth birthday by playing in the local park with his friends. On the positive side, he was perfectly content not celebrating more lavishly. My strokes have forced my two boys to grow up mentally strong, and extremely mature.

In 2024 I moved from my nursing home to a much younger "wheelchair community", and see my kids most weekends. In addition to more traditional physical, occupational & speech therapy, there are lots of music related activities, art and gardening therapy. Plus many outings to choose from. For example: I just returned from a Def Leppard stadium concert, and an excellent private art gallery, both as group outings. I've also performed electric guitar to around 300 people in the resident rock band, which was an epic and exhilarating experience. I'm even learning Italian here! 2024 is definitely the start of my mental and emotional rehabilitation. Obviously stroke is not a desired situation, but I think I've eventually found the facility I was originally meant to be in. My life has seemingly adapted around my abilities, not my disabilities. Today my struggle continues, for tomorrow we fly. ...

5 Vicissitude

Bram Harrison

I stumbled across this word in my eye-controlled computer's predicted text. I'd been given an interest in words because of my need to communicate using alternative methods, due to being non-vocal because of Locked in syndrome (LIS). A Google dictionary search revealed how amazingly well the word fitted my situation:

'Vicissitude'

"A change of circumstances or fortune, typically one that is unwelcome or unpleasant"

My name is Bram. I fractured my skull in a bicycle accident in 1998, resulting in the condition known as 'Locked-in syndrome' (LIS). My brain's motor function is damaged; I'm unable to voluntarily control many of my muscles. However, the intelligent, thinking areas are unaffected.

The condition is described by its name. I am literally locked into most of my body, although parts of me do move. Essentially my eyes. My eyes have replaced my voice and are how I communicate and control the computer that I used to write this chapter.

What follows is an account of some of the more significant points of my Locked-in life. My accident was a split-second event the consequences of which have stolen from every following second.

Expectations, ambitions and dreams, not erased from my memory, just frustratingly from my capability.

Recording information about my individual case of LiS is important. My accident was many years ago, medical practices are updated regularly and vary throughout the world. No two cases are identical, but there are many similarities. If any information about my case of LiS helps somebody in the world make a positive decision regarding LiS, it's been worthwhile.

I've had many different placements into various types of care-setting, with numerous medical professionals, carers/nurses and doctors. Each of these job titles had varying responsibilities within the settings. Each of these settings are run by various organisations. I've deliberately not mentioned specific places.

I was born able-bodied, although I've known people that weren't. Understanding their outlook on life is difficult despite my insight. I've had almost

DOI: 10.4324/9781003464181-5

everything they've never had, taken from me. LiS came later in life due to an accident, an 'acquired brain injury'. Up until ten years old I had a normal English childhood...well, able bodied without major incident and no broken bones etc. Unusual compared to my school friends, many who could boast lists of broken bones, scabby scrapes and the scars of childhood injuries.

I did spend six months of my childhood seeing my mother battling Pancreatic Cancer, after which she sadly passed away. Being so young, it was difficult to comprehend. I remember my school friends talking to me about it and one saying, 'I bet you miss her cooking'. I remember thinking 'how irrelevant'. Now I realise, they were also only little kids.

I don't like talking about Cancer, although I've learnt during my LiS life that discussing difficulties is therapeutic. My mother's case happened thirty years ago. Since then, treatments have improved, and survival rates have increased.

It's always been on my mind. Time has numbed the pain however, Mum will never leave my thoughts. My case of LiS isn't connected, although the feeling of loss is on a devastatingly similar scale. I like to think this painful experience has helped strengthen my resolve throughout the difficulties I've faced during my locked-in years. I've got a self-help audio book about stoicism; I don't think I'll listen to it!

In 1998, I was twenty years old, hardly anybody wore cycling helmets. Over twenty-five years later most people have them and in some countries they are compulsory. Our awareness of the world has increased, changing attitudes for the better. The internet is hugely responsible for this improvement.

Memory and timing escape me. Apparently whilst bike riding with friends. I fell, forehead first onto solid concrete. My brain's jolt inside my skull probably did the damage, although there's no choice about accident types and therefore, I was foolish not to protect the most valuable thing I'll own. Knowing my attitude to life in 1998, I'd say 'I was also, unlucky'

"Hindsight is a beautiful thing."

My accident was sudden; in the tiniest amount of time my life was catastrophically affected. It was a traumatic incident for all involved. Its effects reach beyond me and continue to bite in many ways.

I wasn't aware of it, however inexplicable images have tormented my mind ever since.

I was thankfully with some very good friends when I had the accident, the alternative doesn't bear thinking about. Assisted by some local overnight workers, they got me to hospital, covered with my blood. It must have been horrific.

In the hospital's Accident & Emergency department I was put into a medically induced coma.

My family were contacted; they sat with my comatose body in the hospital's Intensive Care Unit powerless to help. However, just by being there, they were supporting and comforting a brain in turmoil. I regret putting all involved through this experience and testing their commitment to me in such a way. Twenty-five years later my sister among others still helps me. I was at the epicentre of the disaster; however, its aftershocks are continuous and far reaching. Supporting my LiS life has been, and continues to be, a mammoth task, thanks to all involved.

Ever since those first hours, familiar and caring people have been a huge help in my lonely, challenging LiS existence. Do not underestimate the power you're giving someone by just being there.

Apparently shortly afterwards I was transferred to a specialist head injury unit in another hospital in a different city about two hours away.

My Dad, Colin and sister, Emma May, followed the ambulance delivering my comatose body.

I have flickering strands of memory from this time. Describing it coherently is difficult, I've translated many feelings and what I've since understood things to be. I felt a metal object bolted to my skull, a unique and painless sensation. Years later I found out a pressure valve to manage the effects of swelling around my brain was temporarily fitted. Could this object match this mysterious feeling? Hooked up to my ventilator I remember the silence accompanied by lonely darkness, isolated in an inner space with timeless periods of nothing.

The medication was reduced but I didn't respond to early attempts to contact me. I knew people were holding my hand, I remember the instant feeling of comfort this gave me. I saw flickers of vision, my dad's hand holding mine and the hospital blanket.

I was visited by my friend Adam, his mum Tina and sister Leah. They sat with me while my Dad and sister took a much-needed break. I did open my eyes during this time for a few seconds. Apparently, this happened three days after the accident. I had no concept of time.

After this initial memorable encounter with daylight, I opened my eyes regularly when commanded 'open your eyes.' The specialist Doctors decided to send me back to the original hospital. Just before I left the specialist head injury unit, I was told 'when you get outside don't look at the sunshine'. After being trapped in darkness and having this surreal ability to make people happy just by opening my eyes, combined with having the temporary intelligence of a flea, the light was irresistible. Laying on a stretcher opening my eyes whilst gazing skywards was instantly regrettable.

Eventually, I was in familiar surroundings. I vaguely recognised things and gathered I was back in my hometown's hospital. I had the comforting feeling of thinking I was on the home straight; this whole nightmarish situation would soon be over, and I'd be sat at home recovering from my ordeal and preparing to return to work.

If I'd looked down at the mirror image of myself - the beaten up, shell of a human would've been staring back at me - and I'd have realised, I was going nowhere soon, especially not home.

The door and window frames were unique. I could tell I was in a side room of a bigger ward in my local hospital. The area surrounding me was an older part of the hospital which had been rebuilt in the grounds. I had such an intimate understanding of the buildings' architecture because I'd spent a few years selling newspapers to patients and their visitors on the wards of this hospital! I was employed during the transition from old to new buildings. Ominously, I knew these side rooms were reserved for very sick patients, the type that couldn't read newspapers.

Shortly before my consciousness was discovered, my Dad said 'no matter the circumstances, a sign of life means there's hope!' He'd only used such a serious tone in his voice to tell me Mum had terminal cancer. It was then I realised through the confusion, I needed to do something to make people listen. I didn't comprehend my silent and static state. This lack of understanding left me feeling increasingly trapped in a strange isolation. Dad's words inspired me to connect with the doctor.

The Doctor sat beside my bed and said, 'follow my pen with your eyes', he lined it up, so I was looking dead ahead, he slowly raised the pen, my eyes moved upwards accordingly. He repeated similar movements to all four points of the compass to establish the range of movement. His grin said it all. I hadn't reached full range then, however it's improved now. I've since learnt head injuries can restrict the eyes' range of movement.

He explained he was going to give a multiple-choice question, I had to open my eyes when he said my address. When I heard him say 'America Road' my eyes opened, I felt a welcoming warmth like never before. I can remember Dad saying, 'I knew it!'

I noticed some attitudes changing when word got around the hospital wards' staff; 'Bram is in his body'. Looks changed from vacant staring to a smile or a 'hello'. It was like being welcomed back to a place I'd never left. My Dad and sister had always been smiling, I really wanted to tell them how much better my situation was. The peaceful, clear thinking and intelligent mind I enjoy today can safely assume they knew at the time.

With this new ability of saying 'Yes' & 'No', my dad and sister, equipped with determination, pen and paper, developed the 'M' method of communication.

They asked if the letter was a vowel and if not, was it before 'M' in the alphabet, if not after. They would then recite the chosen group of letters until I confirmed with a raised eye the next letter in the word I was communicating.

I can't begin to explain the frustration, but it was all I had so I stuck at it, failure was not an option. It's an incredibly simple and equipment free form of communication when I think about it now.

There seemed to be new faces involved in my care often. Some may have known; however, most were unaware of my communicating ability beyond 'Yes' & 'No'.

The early days in hospital were like repeatedly crawling to hell and back. Progress came in the shape of a ventilator that trained my lungs to work independently. I took my first steps on my mind's unrealistic path home. I've got no recollection of being moved. This tube literally had me by the throat and was pinning me to the bed. I have the greatest respect for people who live on ventilators; it must be incredibly difficult.

I wanted the Tracheostomy tube out of the hole in my neck so I could go home. I was oblivious to the other tubes that continue to sustain my life all these years later. Being paralysed and unable to simply rip the tube out was a blessing in disguise. It would've cut off my air supply, I'd have unwillingly killed myself.

Expectations regarding my future mental state weren't positive from certain medical professionals, it saddens me to think some would've thought of it as the best outcome.

One of the tubes I just mentioned was my original urethral catheter. It blocked for the first time laying relaxed in hospital one evening, in seconds unfamiliar pain surges through me. The same must have happened a thousand times since, however, armed with experience and the ability to communicate effectively, I can deal with it and don't feel like my death is imminent. After years of using different types, I now use a Supra pubic catheter, which takes urine directly from the bladder and quite literally bypasses the middleman. All catheters block and eventually leak - after years of this issue, I've found using purified water beneficial. Everybody's situation is different - follow medical advice that's particularly suited to you.

I can't remember independently breathing for the first time although I can remember coughing and propelling the temporary covering for the hole that medics had cut in my windpipe (trachea) across my hospital room.

At this time, I had little understanding of my own physical state and extremely limited ability. Today, I can easily see the danger, however being inactive for what felt like a lot longer than weeks, simply by coughing I could initiate panicked action. They had to find it, clean it and refit it to my neck, which strangely felt like an achievement. With blind disregard for my own safety, I amused myself a couple of times before a nurse secured it.

Pretending to be emotionally unaffected by something causes stress and unhealthy strain. Admittedly, I learnt this recently and what happened back then was an entirely natural coping system. It wasn't just pain I felt, it was a mental torment on a different scale. My blubbering outpours of emotion mirrored the irregularly spinning ball of confusion exploding in my head on what may have been a daily basis, each time re-forming differently and rarely retaining useful information. It doesn't resemble today's calm intelligence.

Somebody with a greater understanding of what I was going through would have been useful. During my first months of brain injury in 1998, I don't think anyone in my care team had hardly heard of locked in syndrome, let alone had experience of working with someone that had the condition.

Since then, I've heard of an excellent facility in Norway specifically for people diagnosed with LiS. Maybe if a British equivalent existed my life would have been improved. LiS has destroyed my ambitions. I've never realistically replaced them. Maybe creating and living in such a place with my name over the door would be a good one.

I'd been getting out of bed for physio sessions, I'm unsure about how beneficial this was.

On the hospital ward I first experienced a wheelchair!

For able bodied people sitting is a simple exercise.

The reality is you're using secondary muscles in your body you don't even realise you have. When I picture that ward in my mind, it's spinning, like being extremely drunk but with no enjoyment - just endless pressure and stinging pain. The slightest movement meant an increase in painful discomfort. The chair in comparison to modern pressure relieving cushions was prehistoric, I hated it!

The initial hospital stay was four months, I met someone recently that worked with me during this time. She didn't realise at first how my mentality had changed; she described me as being grumpy. I'd describe my mood back then as the lowest of the low, way below grumpy!

After a long wait suffering the inescapable hustle and bustle of the hospital ward I moved into the sanctuary of the rehabilitation unit.

My mental energy was draining because of the confusion, fear and worry. I told myself in the peaceful rehabilitation unit, this is no way forward. I had learnt harshly in other upsetting times; tears don't bring anything back.

I won't let not eating depress me. It seems that would be an easy trap to fall into. Seeing mouthwatering TV food adverts for this many years and knowing the reality is that it'd be very harmful for me (i.e. I couldn't chew and swallow without choking), naturally has lessened the blow of my brain's food desires. However, people discussing food triggers painful memories which often come back to haunt me when I'm hungry.

Physically I eat "artificially"; I don't experience the taste and texture of food. I do get the feeling of having a full stomach, but it leaves me naturally as digestion occurs. The liquid food gets gently pumped into my stomach three times a day, using a drip pump. Similar systems deliver intravenous or IV medication to the body, it's Latin for Into the Vein. The liquid food goes through a surgically cut hole in my stomach wall and through a Percutaneous endoscopic gastrostomy (PEG) tube.

I've had two of these surgically cut, the first must have been shortly after the accident, it got re-sited due to tissue weakness. It was painless, although tender for months after. If it's not prodded or pulled, I can live with it.

I'd describe what I eat as a litre of UHT milk, with all the nutrients and goodness a human requires to survive liquidised into the mixture. It resembles the exact colour of a milky cup of tea. A previous carer experienced the flavour when he left a cup of tea in my bedroom as he left for a toilet break.

With my permission another carer poured a mouthful of my feed onto the top of his tea. On his return, I was barely holding in my hysterics as he picked up the cup. I think his last words were 'What's the matter with Bram?' before taking a swig and then instantly propelling the contents of his mouth across my room, followed by the cry of 'YOU BASTARDS!!'... Apparently, it's quite a sour taste!

I've digested several swimming pools worth of this liquid food, it contains nothing but nutrients and goodness, so I was confident a mouthful wouldn't harm him. The victim was fine and laughing about his traumatic taste experience like a victorious hero.

I don't think anybody brought a cup of tea into my room again.

PEG tubes have come a long way in twenty-five years. An earlier type that was designed to last a few years broke down and corroded internally and had to be replaced. I hate the long-lasting type, they get filthy.

I now use a balloon gastrostomy tube. It's like what I had before, although it can be changed without going to hospital. I used to endure an overnight stay followed by general anaesthetic in the morning every few years for twenty-five years. So much hassle, the development is amazing.

I've attempted to eat several times; controlling anything that moves faster in my mouth than thick yoghurt is uncomfortably dangerous. I've aspirated things before, it's painful and frightening.

I've no swallow reflex, it's a perfect example of "you don't know what you've got till it's gone".

My Speech and Language Therapist, Gill Hardy, showed me a communication device called an 'E-trans board', which at first looked incredibly complicated. However, I learnt the technique, it was simple.

Look at the direction my eye points through the hole in the middle of the board. Ask for a corner, then colour. The letter = the colour of the letter in my chosen corner. I'll give you a 'yes' or 'no' eye signal after each corner, colour and letter choice. Always write down the letters. Words will appear, after a few letters you can make a sensible guess what the word will be e.g., HAV - have, CAT - catheter. It looks a lot more complicated in writing than in practice.

Although my up and down eye movements were fine, I struggled to point them left and right. I can remember the fuzzy boarded vision, although the improvement to my sights' capabilities today was so gradual it's difficult to gauge. My extremely limited neck control is another area where paralysis has been a blessing in disguise. I think it's compensated by improving the range of my eyeball's movement, although I'm sure other factors have contributed.

The power of communication for paralysed people is truly awesome and would've also been a big draw.

The more that a carer is involved with my care, the greater their knowledge and ease of this skill.

In my locked-in speechless life, all my carers need to use it. I rely on it during personal care, at night and any time I'm away from my Hi-Tech talking eye-controlled computer.

Roughly two hundred people have learnt how to use my board. They were of all ages; the youngest was five years old. Everyone has varying abilities, and none have been good straight away. Everyone makes mistakes - they learn and in their own time they improve. I've never known a newborn talking baby!

My eye pointing letter board has been a vital tool easing many difficult situations, helping to make my LiS life bearable.

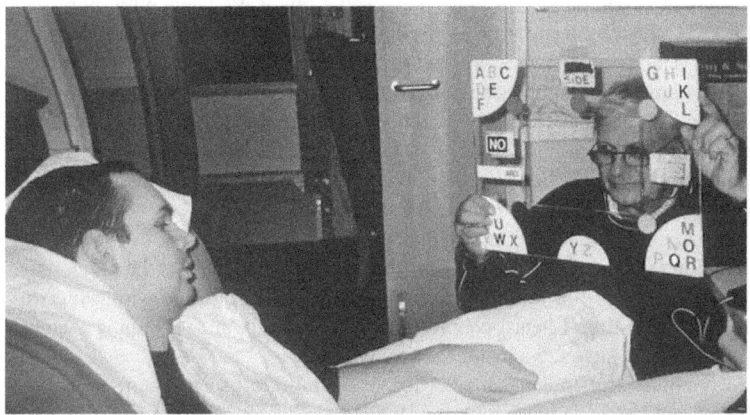

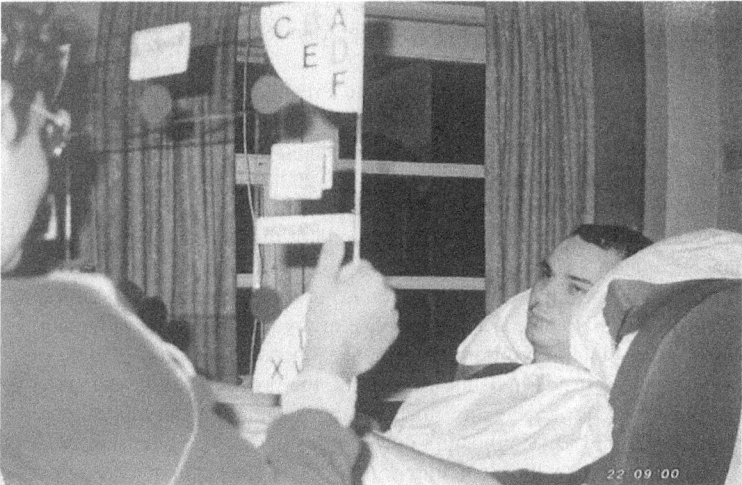

Figures 5.1 and 5.2 E-Trans communication with my father and sister.

I need the reassurance of continuity of care. My life is incredibly difficult after being rocked by a devastating event which disrupted every normality I've known since birth. I need the same people doing the same things day after day; predictability and routine needs to replace everything. Explaining something to a different person every time adds to my frustration. My most effective carers know my complex way of life completely. They work with me regularly.

In the hospital room, a computer was brought in. I couldn't interface with it; this was years before eye control. It was disappointingly wheeled out the next day.

My next computer encounter happened a few years later. With more success. My Dad built me a PC; I used a blink switch and operated a program called 'Hands off'. It was written by 'Sensory software', which later became 'Smart box' - a computer company that's helped me throughout my LiS life.

I couldn't get my wheelchair close to the monitor. Some friends raised funds to buy me a huge screen - it cost thousands - today the same can be purchased for a few hundred. The switch became difficult to use, and I had to give up, it's different from modern eye control.

Listening to the radio during the day broke the monotony of watching TV, only long enough for the same tactic to work in reverse against the radio. After ten years of my life failing to improve, the positive attitude within me was fading. Each time I heard people around me were doing something vaguely interesting, it gave me a jealous crushing feeling.

A university student called Alice learnt how to use my communication board and began to work with me. We created a 'My space' account... yeah that long ago! Alice and Gill assisted me to trial five eye-controlled devices, the 'Tobi-I P10', using operating software from 'Smart box' was a clear winner. I've had a few new computers since.

The eye-controlled computer gave me a revolutionary grasp of the world and it's grown with my ability. At last, I could control the TV and my wall-to-wall collection of VHS tapes, (considered a major fire risk it was so stacked!). Now modern video streaming sites have solved that issue.

Above all, initiating conversation with a clear message using my own word choice felt fantastic. It was easily one of the best things that has ever happened in my LiS life.

An annoying trait of ECC, however, is not being able to respond instantly when spoken to. People that are unaware of my restrictions leave feeling ignored. To maintain my optimum computer operating position is to stay focused on the screen's invisible sweet spot, the precise area the computer is using infrared to track the movement of my eyeball. You can trigger a previously written message, although I only use this in certain circumstances.

My low-tech spelling communication board doesn't require me to use complete and correct spellings.

After nine years of relying entirely on my spelling board for communication, the skills needed to build words, sentences and paragraphs coherently were gone, leaving me with a jumbled mess. The ECC gave me the ability to write, but no vital text construction skills.

The technology was in its infancy. Early attempts at a coherent message were juvenile. What happened next helped kick start my brain…

I'll never forget when Philip Robinson said, 'great Email, you're actually starting to use punctuation and paragraphs like an adult'. Phil then introduced me to his friend Tony Walker; he had an interest in computers and would like to see the technology that I used. I met Tony a few times and he started to build what is now my website, not easily done back then. Knowing about my interest in music and especially DJ-ing which my accident curtailed, they developed the idea of me producing a radio show, assisted by them (with regards to the technological limitations back then).

Although I'd been involved in some very minor creative music projects with Phil, I'd not produced anything that left my room. I had no doubt - I was determined to make it work!

Using the alias 'Dj Eye Tech', I wrote and presented with my eye-controlled computer sixteen, two-hour long shows between 2012 & 2014. I made a shorter charity show several years later. During the shows' lifetime I played over two hundred different songs. OK, a couple were repeated, however that's not bad considering it wasn't generally mainstream recordings. Music was different - we've been through a Digital music revolution - online archives existed. However, their variety was limited, my multi-genre show was hardly catered for and missed out.

Naming the show was simple. I had the song lyric, 'Let me walk you through the corridors of My Life!' running around in my head. 'My life' soon became 'Eye life'.

The earlier shows used ET's movie theme. I then saw a repeated episode of the 1960's TV show 'The Prisoner' (definitely a repeat) with dramatic countdown to transmission and punchy tune. I wrote a boxer's style ring announcement, Phil adopted a dodgy accent and performed like Michael Buffer the second.

The show was Internet based, as well as its local broadcast on Phonic FM. This was a few years before the DAB days. I was receiving just as many global emails as from local listeners. Naturally, the International Eye Life show was born.

It's said "sometimes rock bottom is your trampoline" I've come back from that place. Strangers would say I'm still there, however emerging from comatose darkness to the very conscious and intelligent mental state I enjoy today has been an incredible achievement. Something within the overall accomplishment was writing and presenting with my eye-controlled computer The International Eye Life radio show.

The ECC I used predated Microsoft Windows and even then, had limited abilities within its eye-controlled scope. It was, though, a state-of-the-art system, despite being frustratingly unforgiving after the slightest mistake. Today the ECC I'm using runs Grid 3, from the Smart box company and controls Microsoft Windows 10. I enjoy having virtually total computer control, everything works so much more smoothly. Given the opportunity again, writing my Eye Life radio shows in the same way on modern ECC's would be easy.

The radio show gave me a sense of achievement beyond the daily grind of living with LiS; for the first time since that night in 1998, it provided other opportunities. I made two television appearances, one of which was shown in many other countries. I expect I was the first person to swear on UK TV using an eye-controlled computer.

I featured in the national press, where I opposed a ridiculous attempt to change UK law to allow assisted suicide for people with LiS. Euthanasia for other things is a very difficult subject. Blurring the clear line between life and death would be dangerous, vulnerable voiceless minorities must be protected.

Most people in the UK are really accommodating of my disability. After a music concert, a total stranger cleared a path through a crowd of ninety thousand hyped Foo-fighter fans as my sister pushed my wheelchair through the dense forest of legs to the car park outside. This guy's efforts to negotiate with countless people to shuffle out of my way made a bad situation bearable. I have encountered a few idiots in the public. One was Julian, on a mission from God to get me walking ASAP. I was laughing so much, I triggered some Clones in my arms, it's a painless involuntary muscle spasm, look it up? After seeing this movement Julian started to believe his own bullshit as his wife dragged him away. There's been whispering and staring but this doesn't bother me. Random acts of kindness by far out way the thoughtless few.

Several years ago, a friend I'd made since my accident asked me if I knew a certain person from before the acquired brain injury and subsequent years of LiS. The person in question was someone I knew from my able-bodied teenage years. They were having a conversation, and I was mentioned, both realised they had a mutual friend. Although the first friend said they'd been told I'd died in hospital. I've heard similar stories from other friends. I feel during my very internal battles with my own mind, I've drawn energy from my memories of good times spent with these people. It's sad to think they no longer thought I existed. This is one of those many times I've looked up and thought, why?

Trying to remember things has been difficult because for years I've rejected these painful memories.

Being disabled has opened my eyes to aspects of health and life. Some people's preconceptions about disability are ill-thought and ridiculous. Before my accident, I had some ignorant views about disability that with my insight now, are too embarrassing to mention.

6 Locked Out

A Real-Life Story

Dick van der Heijde

As a locked-in individual, I feel quite locked out. In fact, my struggle for recognition began when I slowly regained consciousness after a brainstem stroke mercilessly struck me down on the night of August 31, 1991, at the age of 28. That stroke was caused by a nasty clump of cholesterol that had blocked the blood flow to my brain in a rather unfortunate location.

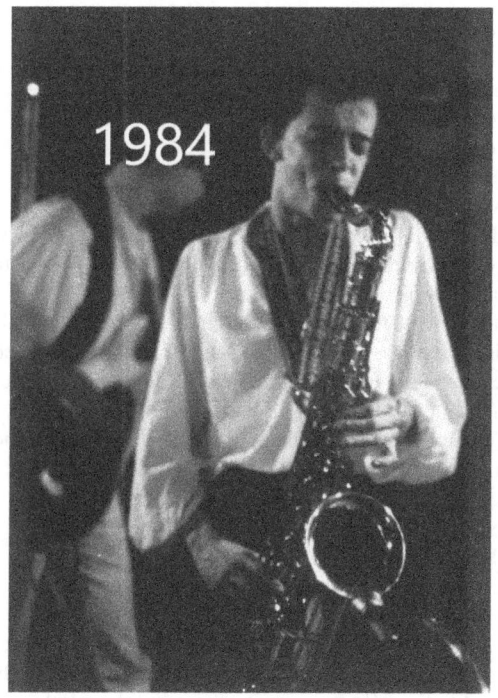

Figure 6.1 Photo of me and my passion.

DOI: 10.4324/9781003464181-6

There you are, a thinking do-nothing, completely paralyzed, slightly spastic, and deprived of my ability to speak. The surroundings of my hospital room in Goes, which is located in the South-West of the Netherlands, were not really great either. A desire for self-assertion has never been foreign to me since birth. The urge to create something has been a common thread throughout my life. I took great pleasure in playing the saxophone in various bands for many years. Making music and expressing my feelings were my passion and my life. From the day I became locked-in, that need turned into an urgency. It began more or less on the day they taught me how to communicate. Who spells "quasar" as their first word? I do.

The first few days in the ICU were quite bizarre for my family, not for me, because I lay there like a sleepy rabbit in dreamland. Sometimes, I had to cough so hard I sat up in bed due to the power of my back muscles. It must have looked like a scene from a horror movie. Gradually, I became more aware of reality, and in due course, I saw things as they were. My family had noticed I could consciously blink my eyes and had conveyed that to the nursing staff. They then promptly conducted a brilliant test with me. One by one, a member of the nursing staff entered my room with a question.

"Do I have red hair?"

"Do I have black hair?"

"Am I blonde?"

"Do I have long hair?"

"Do I have curly hair?"

"Do I wear glasses?"

"Am I a woman?"

Again and again I blinked once for yes and twice for no, as we had agreed. I got it right every time, and so the conclusion was drawn I could hear, see, and think clearly. I was then showered with affection.

From that moment, the focus was entirely on communication. Initially, they tried using a device, but because I saw all its lights jumbled up, I knew within two seconds it wouldn't work. The next day, an occupational therapist and a speech therapist attempted an auditory approach, which worked like a charm. Let me explain. The principle is childishly simple. The alphabet is divided into three rows.

1st row: a b c d e f g h i
2nd row: j k l m n o p q r
3rd row: s t u v w x y z

Someone asks; "1st row, 2nd row, 3rd row?" When they reach the correct row, I blink, and then they recite the letters in that row. When they reach the correct letter, I blink again, and we continue until the whole word is spelled out. It's painstaking, but it's working well.

What I found exceptionally pleasant was the doctor allowed me to choose from five rehabilitation centers where I wanted to go. That was truly an outstanding treatment. As an adult, I spent seven months in a children's rehabilitation center on the Veluwe, the woody heart of the Netherlands. If there's one thing that's good for your self-esteem, it's being around children. After a brief transitional period in a nursing home, I was brought into our new house on November 20, 1992. Our house, because my then-girlfriend and I looked forward to the future together with confidence.

She had tastefully decorated the house, although it must be said I had frequently given my opinions and advice on the colors. What immediately caught my eye when she wheeled me in were two columns filled with all my CDs (there were about fifty at that time). It surprises me I thought I had such a large collection back then. Currently, it's 80 times larger.

The first ten years of my new life had two enormous milestones. The first was the birth of our son Owen in 1999, but honestly, witnessing his growth was continuously fantastic. The other highlight was the publication of my first book and everything that came with it. Need for self- assertion? The Province of Zeeland provided a massive grant so we could give 'M'n Ogen Zeggen Alles' ('My Eyes Tell It All') a splendid presentation. It's indescribable what feelings went through me on that day.

Through the book (or, more precisely, the manuscript), I got in touch with two filmmakers who eventually made a 50-minute TV documentary about our family. It greatly stroked my ego the viewership ratings were so good. Hundreds of thousands of people watched the broadcast. Among them was Maarten, the founder of 'Progwereld'. That's a website about progressive rock, my favorite music genre. He asked if I wanted to write columns for his site, which turned into a 19-year collaboration in which I reviewed approximately 600 CDs. I also got in touch with Herman, an IT specialist who wanted to help me find the right speech adaptation. I almost immediately convinced him I needed a custom program. The letters had to be large and appear one at a time on the screen. With the regular adaptations, I was presented with the entire alphabet at once, which I couldn't work with. I physically can't read because the brainstem stroke also paralyzed the muscles that allow me to move my eyes sideways. For this reason, I asked Herman to equip the program with a scrollbar so I could constantly see the sentences I created moving from right to left across the screen. Picture it like a red bar above a butcher's counter, showcasing the pork chops. And that's how it happened I've been sitting behind SIDE every day for more than twenty years, writing at my own pace. Another viewer of our real-life documentary was a 14-year-old boy who was inspired to write a song. Roel wrote it as part of the national Junior Song Festival. He made it through round after round, had the song professionally recorded, and ultimately won the final. Since then, there's been a gap in the wall, and Roel travels the world as a celebrated musical artist.

But as for my relationship with my girlfriend, we were always good, and even in the first ten years after my stroke, everything was hallelujah. Over time, things began to shift, which culminated in a divorce in 2006. Where there's a divorce, there's always a lot of bickering. My goodness, was I going to run the show by myself now? In that regard, the feelings I had after the divorce were as genuine as they could be. I always saw the fact I was on my own as a tremendous challenge I was eager to take on. I set new goals for myself, new projects.

There was a long road ahead of me.

"That didn't take away the fact that my mind had to anticipate the processing of all those changes for the second time. My dreams often revolved around being lost. In my subconscious, I was repeatedly directed to a pier with the sea as the endpoint. Sometimes you just have to be your own psychologist, even if it's from scratch."

From the very beginning of our plans to get divorced it was immediately clear that Owen would go with his mother. We didn't even really discuss it. For me that was just logical and I was sure she would raise him wonderfully. That turned out to be true, Owen has grown into a great guy with a good job, a beautiful house nearby and a lovely girlfriend he's been living with for years.

I am naturally excessively positive, and after my stroke, that positivity only intensified, as if I had to use my optimistic mindset. What helped me a lot was I was in a positive flow right from the beginning in the ICU. Everyone was super nice and, above all, very dedicated. My rehabilitation doctor took the lead in that regard, but the occupational therapist, the speech therapist, the social worker, and the various physiotherapists were also my best friends. Not very sympathetic, however, was my neurologist. Much to the anger of my girlfriend, he refused to tell me what had happened to me. Another neurologist recognized the issue and offered to help with our case. He was a great guy who suggested applying cotton swabs with whisky to my tongue. Now that got my attention. Most of the positivity, of course, came from my family and friends who fully embraced who I was. I call myself nauseatingly positive; there was nothing fake about it.

A helper, let's call her Anja, saw my marriage falling apart and offered to help me. She did a good job. Even before the year ended, she managed to have me reevaluated as a single person and also enrolled me with a care agency, which led to one fine day in December when ten brand-new caregivers came over for coffee. What a luxury! Well, it wasn't all that. Anja didn't get along well with one of the coordinators from the care agency. Creating a cohesive schedule was always a problem, and because Anja often got furious on the phone, she was forbidden from interfering with the schedule any longer. Anja had a fitting countermeasure, one I fully agreed with. She asked all the caregivers if they wanted to work directly under me.

I was quite pleased with that, as the care agency charged a significant amount as mediation fees from my PGB (an allowance from health insurance to pay caregivers). Anja and I agreed I would complete 90 percent of the schedules, and she would fill in the remaining gaps. That worked perfectly, but as Anja started to behave more bossy, friction arose, and Anja put herself on leave. There was another caregiver who wanted to take over her duties. It didn't take long because I ended up in the hospital with double pneumonia, and nobody had any idea how to handle the financial aspect of it. There was only one thing to do…call Anja and ask her to help us, and so the boomerang came back.

2013 was an eventful year for me, and it began in the spring. An editor from the TV show 'De Reünie' (The Reunion) asked if I was interested in participating in their program. She had found me through a mutual contact, the filmmaker of the documentary. I didn't waste any time and quickly sent an email back. A week later, we were already sitting around the table to discuss everything. It turned into a beautiful episode where I went to see my favorite band, which played a song I had composed in the 80s. The emotionally charged conversation about relationships presenter Rob Kamphues had with me also made a deep impression. It's worth giving the director a big compliment when you see how well the other stories in the program are blended. The episode provides a perfect picture of that afternoon in the school desks at the Media Park in Hilversum.

A pleasant consequence of my participation in the program was that Rob and I became friends afterward. I was supposed to visit him with a Facebook friend at the Zandvoort circuit, but at the time, I started having breathing issues and was permanently on oxygen. They prefer not to see you on the circuit when you're like that. What a shame.

Meanwhile, things weren't going well on the home front either. Anja became more bossy and dominant, and everyone had to bear the brunt of it. She scolded me several times, furious and absolutely overstepping boundaries. The most embarrassing tirade I ever received from her was in the hospital corridor. It was teeming with people, a reason for her to lash out even more fiercely. There was really nothing wrong. The day before, it was touch-and-go whether I could end my stay in the ICU that evening or the next morning. A nurse came to inform me. "We think it's better for you to go home tomorrow morning," he explained. I didn't even think about it; Anja would already know, she was on top of everything. An hour later, the phone rang, it was Anja asking if I knew anything yet. When she heard that I had been aware for an hour that I couldn't go home that day, she became furious with me, and she repeated it the next day in the corridor while waiting for the taxi. She could also be quite nice and good. We would play music by Caravan or Jethro Tull, and then she would be in her element. She often talked about the trouble she had with others and how I was her easiest client, although she did have control of my bank card, not with the intention of taking my money, by the way.

That year also saw three hospitalizations due to respiratory problems and, as a result, a fourth to insert a tracheostomy tube. A what??? A tracheostomy tube. A hole was made at the level of my Adam's apple, leading into my airpipe. This cavity houses the tracheostomy tube. Through this artificial opening, my caregivers can clean my airways of mucus with a small tube. Of course, they can't do it just like that; they first had to undergo training at the

CTB (Center for Home Ventilation). It's quite a hassle, but it's effective. Anja arranged for three ICU nurses from the area to be here daily to oversee everything. Given their job, they were also authorized to evaluate the caregivers on behalf of the CTB. This all got even more complicated when I started night ventilation about a month later. It's a mecca of tubes and hoses here; I have them in all shapes and sizes. Try to make sense of it all.

For Anja, all these measures were a reason to tighten the screws even more. She became ultra-strict, not only with me; most of the helpers were reduced to tears by the director. She constantly quarreled with two (good) caregivers. She couldn't fire them, so her trick was not to schedule them anymore.

We were in an atmosphere where I began to dislike her, and then Billy joined the team. Billy was very nice during her first few shifts, but I have never seen anyone provoke so much antipathy as she did. I hoped I would find an ally in Anja, but unfortunately, the opposite was true. Billy started doing substitute work for Anja's company and was favored in every way. What an incredibly manipulative pair of know-it-alls. And they could humiliate. The saddest thing Billy ever said: "You pay me a presence fee, and for that money, you entertain yourself." Here's another gem from her to her colleagues: "You have to realize he has a brain injury and is no longer 100 percent."

Saturday, July 7, 2018, was a memorable day for me, or to use a title from Pink Floyd: "A Great Day For Freedom." In the morning, Billy resigned, and around lunchtime, Anja came. She had brought her husband Hans with her to reinforce her resignation. Why so intimidating, Anja? Hans snapped at me I had ruined his vacation and banged on the table. Well, Hans, I thought, you have your lovely wife to thank for that. She has conflicts with so many people; it's only natural someone starts a legal process against her. Don't blame me for that. Anja made a move to leave, put on her coat, and left. She hadn't even left the garden path when I rushed to the computer to copy our shared Dropbox with all vital information about my care. My premonition told me she was going to delete it, and yes... a day later, everything was gone except for my copy, of course. I never saw her again.

One evening, the doorbell rang at my parents' house. It was Hans. Without saying a word, he handed over a full bag and left as silently as he had come. Once in the living room, my parents opened the bag to see what was inside. It was full of various items related to my care, like a needle container, a few syringes, an empty medication dispenser, some notebooks, etc. It was a good thing my parents inspected it all the way to the bottom because there, right at the very bottom was (you won't believe it)... my bank card. Real professional, Anja.

Christel, a great caregiver of mine, had been working on scheduling several weeks before Anja left. One thing led to another, and in no time Christel was fully trained in the administrative side of my care. Unfortunately, it was a shame for Christel she had to deal with a pitifully low hourly wage we could afford to pay the caregivers. This made it increasingly difficult to keep the team at full strength. Whenever people left, we had to search high and low for replacements.

It didn't get any better, and the sad part was no one was to blame. It was what it was. My motto closely aligned with Christel's. Just try to make the best of it.

Meanwhile, I was busy writing my second book, which was to be titled 'What It's Like Being My Parents'. I wanted to describe my youth and also had a strong desire to thank my parents for their wonderful upbringing. The writing itself went smoothly, and finding a publisher was a breeze. A friend of mine had taught for years and had become a language purist par excellence, the perfect person to proofread my work. We spent months dotting the i's and crossing the t's. Behind the scenes, I was busy organizing a book launch. I made every effort to have it held at 't Beest, a youth center in Goes where I used to go often. I wanted Rob Kamphues to present the evening; his humor would fit well with what I had in mind. Rob was on the other side of the world when I emailed him, but eventually, I managed to get him on the stage of 't Beest on the evening of October 17, 2019. I was incredibly lucky because everyone I wanted to invite could actually make it that night, from the cameraman to the book saleswoman, and from Roel, who sang his song festival song, to Christel in her lilac outfit. It became the night of my life, and I couldn't care less I had to dig deep into my pockets to cover all the costs. I was proud of everything and everyone, my family, my caregivers, and my friends. What a stroke of luck Christel had dressed me up in a fancy tuxedo that night.

Christel and I had discovered a website where you could buy international second-hand CDs, like a marketplace for music. We would often spend hours on the computer searching for interesting albums. I ordered hundreds of copies from places like Brazil, Taiwan, Spain, Finland, and even from Russia (back then it was still possible). I ordered CDs from Italy, Bulgaria, Canada, Australia, you name it. Christel knew the program inside out, and so did I.

The reason I'm such a huge music fan (and still am) is because it was ingrained in me from an early age. My father enrolled me in the local fanfare when I was only six years old, and he played in it himself. My mother, on the other hand, was less musically inclined, but she worked in a store that also sold records and would frequently buy singles for me. I received my first saxophone when I was 12, and from then on, I was hooked. The great thing about a saxophone is every music group has a place for the instrument. What was clear to me was that, due to the stroke, I was completely "unsaxed." To be of any significance, I would have to fully utilize my taste and knowledge of music.

I had been living at home for just over a year when I was already asked to write reviews. At that time, I corresponded a lot with various musicians and read everything I could find about my favorite music genre. Word quickly spread even in the pre-Facebook era.

One thing led to another and in 2002 I joined the 'Progwereld' team. Over the years, I saw that Maarten's website was visited by millions of readers each year. There was no way I would ever leave that club. However, it did happen. I desperately felt the need to have a place of my own. No more reviewing the latest albums, just CDs from my own collection. Together with Elbert, one of my caregivers, I built a website. It was a tough job as neither of us had any experience with it. I feel immensely proud of what we have achieved, and I'm fiercely passionate about 'www.progenrock.com'.

And then there was also something called coronavirus. Initially, I was quite afraid of losing acquaintances to the disease. That never happened in the end. I only know a few people who actually experienced problems from it. There was a lot of fearmongering. What I did find strange was how people dealt with the concept of a 'lockdown.' Well, I've been living in lockdown for thirty years, so don't whine when you can't go to the pub for a few months. There was, however, a legitimate concern I might contract the virus... and sure enough, in March 2022, I was infected. The self-test turned positive within five seconds, but I actually knew it before that. My ventilation machine was on continuously from then on, and because I was frequently suctioned, I was rid of my sore throat within a few days. It hurt so much when they used the suction tube, but complaining is not in my vocabulary.

Although staff shortages in healthcare have been an issue for years, during the coronavirus crisis, it was like trying to bail out a sinking ship with a bucket. My work schedule was a worrisome Swiss cheese, and a consultant from the CTB (Center for Home Ventilation) stepped in. On July 12, 2022, I was admitted to the ICU in Goes, completely healthy. It was embarrassing. Thanks to the efforts of a large number of stakeholders who seriously pulled some strings, I was allowed to go home five weeks later. The sun had started shining for me again because a cry for help on Facebook and regional, even national publicity had brought me in contact with about thirty potential new caregivers, and some former helpers had also decided to rejoin the team.

Just before I went to the ICU, Christel had brought her daughter along. I had met Michelle a few times before, but it took at least half an hour before I realized who she was. It was funny she was interested in working with me. During her first one-on-one interaction, we talked about TikTok, and during her training at the ICU, we brainstormed further. In the meantime, we have a highly successful account with over 20,000 followers, about 100,000 likes, and a tremendous number of views on our videos. Every Wednesday night, we go live to chat with our viewers about Locked-In Syndrome. The most frequently asked question to Michelle is, "What's wrong with your father?"

One afternoon in the ICU, my brother came by. He had brought our mother with him, and I was so proud of her. Alzheimer's had certainly flattened her personality, but her sweet character was lovelier than ever. My mother and I had that typical mother-son relationship. She was always there for me, and I for her. Along with my father, she sat by my bedside for hours in the months after my stroke. She took a taxi every two weeks to Arnhem to pick me up when I was on weekend leave from the rehabilitation center. She was distraught. She cried her heart out completely, over and over again... That afternoon, Michelle saw her for the first and last time. A few weeks later, my dear mother passed away from kidney failure. I wrote a song lyric for her.

So Red The Rose

> So red the rose, so
> dark the night I'm looking
> through your eyes
> Your hands are mine
> We changed the colors many times
> But never in this way
> Why did your mind turn so white?
> We didn't need to step to align
> We already were
> We didn't have to try
> It all was clear
> Right from the start
> Right from the start
> Out of tears you were
> Did I put you through?
> We are riding cross the rainbow
> Where even angels dare to fly
> Carry on
> Carry on
>   © Dick van der Heijde 2022

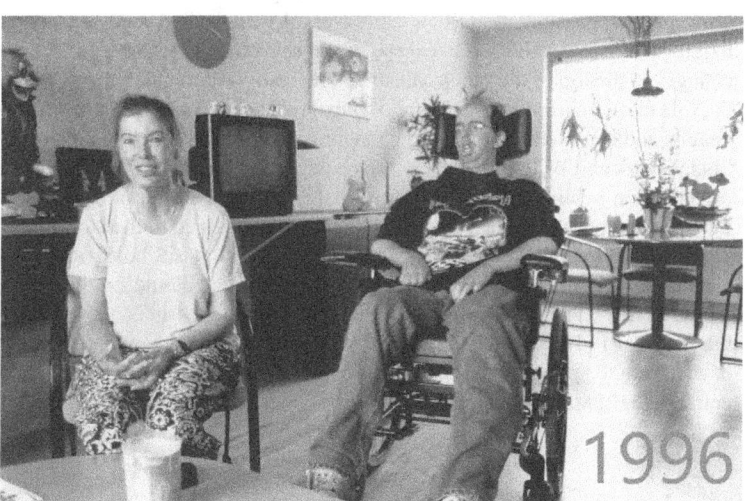

Figure 6.2 Photo of me and my mum.

In the years when Mom was overwhelmed by her dementia, Dad showed exceptional care. Beautiful, of course, except he eventually sank into a persistent depression. Brother Marco had a full-time job keeping everything on track, but he succeeded brilliantly. When Mom passed away, things really went downhill for Dad. He was completely apathetic and suffered from epileptic seizures. After several weeks in the hospital, he ended up in a psychiatric care facility, where he miraculously recovered quickly. Marco managed to secure a spot for him in a brand-new nursing home in the city center of Goes. He enjoys it there immensely, and Marco and I, along with the rest of the family, are as happy as can be. We have our dad back. Yay!

Amidst all these hyper-emotional moments, there were also a few bright spots. Every Wednesday evening the local radio station of Friesland, located on the other side of the Netherlands, plays a song I've selected. The presenter is my age, and we both love music from the 70s in our own way. She leans more towards country, while my heart beats faster for progressive rock. There is indeed an overlap, or to put it in the title of her program: we both have a lot of 'Leafde Foar Muzyk' ('Love For Music').

Also, I was asked to give a course on locked-in syndrome as an experiential expert at the HAN (Hogeschool Arnhem Nijmegen). That was right up my alley, as I had studied at the PABO for two years in the 80s. Together with some assistants, I created a PowerPoint presentation and arranged for two nurses to help me share my story online. For someone with spasticity, it was incredibly nerve-wracking. My muscle relaxant was my best friend.

The nicest bright spot was things were going really well with my team. The health insurance had roughly doubled my budget, and I could hire a whole army of young, enthusiastic new caregivers. I was thrilled, and I no longer had to worry about the Swiss cheese of the schedule. This did lead to some changes in the top of the 'Dick Management Team.' Marco was appointed for the role of guaranteed assistance, and an external agency was brought in for financial and contractual matters, in collaboration with SMWO (Foundation for Social Work and Welfare in the OosterscheldVeregio), in order to have a neutral organization behind me. This meant Christel's role took a bit of a back seat, but it never caused any real friction. She now has returned to the workplace.

Recently, I was asked to write my life story for this LiS book. It became clear to me right away that my desire for recognition should be the central theme of it all. The total number of years I've been locked-in is dominated by the fact that I always have to prove myself. Well, I would say there's plenty of evidence to support that. I've enjoyed revisiting the past, and I've actually come to the same conclusion for years: I'd rather be here than not.

7 I'm Still Here

Ann Johnson

My journey started on February 14, 2005. I had no warning signs except a prolonged cold which is not strange for January in Canada. I was 30, was not a smoker, rarely drank. I had low blood pressure, was fit, not on birth control and had given birth 13 months earlier. I had a vertebral dissection which caused a pooling of blood in the brainstem which then caused a brainstem stroke. Doctors have never known why I had the stroke but I like to believe I was born with a weak spot on my artery. I was so angry for the first few years, then started thinking; thank goodness it was me and not one of my friends. I have an extremely supportive family, I'm from a country with universal health care, I belong to a union and still get paid 70% of my wage each month and my union had disability insurance for me.

The day of my stroke was just like any other day. My husband, Bill, left for work and I got myself and baby daughter ready for the day. I went to my parent's farm just outside the city, left our daughter with them then headed to the high school in the city I taught at. I taught all day and felt fine. At the end of the school day I met my husband and daughter in my office. I will forever remember the smile on my daughter's face when she saw me that day. From there Bill went to coach basketball and my daughter and I headed to the art room. We spent about an hour helping students decorating the gym for an upcoming basketball tournament. Then we got groceries, met my husband at home and he cooked supper. I swung by the high school to help with the decorating then headed to my ladies' volleyball league; that is where the event happened.

There were 6 of us and we were warming up for the game when I felt dizzy like I had never been before. I alerted my friends somehow because they helped me safely to the floor. I kept saying it would go away, but it never did. I remember watching a friend call 911 while another cradled my head in her lap. Everyone was holding my hand or leg. At this point my brain started to accept that there was something wrong. The paramedics were just a few blocks away and came quickly.

When the paramedics got there, I started to throw up and wondered if I had food poisoning. One of the EMTs got me talking and I was beginning to slur; I realized I was having a stroke. I started to relax because I thought a mystery

DOI: 10.4324/9781003464181-7

had been solved in my mind. I remember seeing that the EMTs had a trainee with them. He was so nervous and I remember feeling bad for him. I don't remember how I got on the stretcher but I remember being put in the ambulance on a cold February night, I was in shorts and a t-shirt and the cold winds crept up my blankets. In the ambulance I felt calm and relaxed; I remember the EMT talking to me reassuringly. To that point in my life, I had never felt a person's energy, but I felt his. I felt myself fading but I truly didn't care. I remember telling myself that I was about to die, and I didn't care. I simply faded to black.

Much to my surprise, I woke up to the noise of the overhead heaters in the ambulance bay. It was here that confusion, hallucination and dreams mixed with reality. I don't remember much of the ER, but I do remember an Asian male nurse. The main memory was my husband coming into the room. Sometimes I feel tingly and happy when I see him, but this was not one of those times. My first thought was where is the baby! Next, I reminded myself that it would be silly to take a 13-month-old to the ER. I found myself feeling shame that I was here and injured. Over the next 10 years there were a lot of feelings of shame and guilt.

I have no clear memories of the next 24 hours. I find that a lot of my hospital memories are audio. It must take a lot less energy for the brain to store audio memories then visual ones. I remember that at this time I could still talk and could move my right side. I remember my mother-in-law crying and some co-workers dropping by with cookies. I was told I had a stroke but that I wouldn't hold still for my MRI so they couldn't tell me where the stroke was in the brain. I remember waking up in the MRI tube, those noises totally freaked me out!

That night I was on an acute ward. Bill was strongly encouraged to go home, eat, play with the baby and sleep. Later that night I remember waking up and gasping for breath, hearing lots of voices and someone trying to intubate me. It took 3 tries, I remember all of it. Again, I had no energy to panic, I quietly lay there hoping it would get done. When COVID hit I was reliving that trauma every day when the number of people intubated was announced. PTSD is not only present in those that go to war.

I spent about a month in the ICU. My main memory of the ICU was that a former student's sister was a nurse there. She got me the best things she could, read me her son's travel journal and simply cared for me. My body temperature was affected by the stroke so I was often very hot, there was always a large fan pointed at me. Everyday a portable x-ray was taken of my lungs to check for pneumonia, I loved to experience that cool board being slipped under my back. An ICU nurse taught me to blink once for yes, twice for no.

70-80% of the time that I was in the ICU, I spent dreaming and hallucinating. There was one I had a lot and I have flashbacks of it. I am at the top of the Eiffel Tower, and I fell off. I fell for days and never hit the ground. Before the stroke I had no fear of heights, but I do now.

My family was told I would very likely die; there was brain activity but not much. I couldn't even close my eyes for the first 2 weeks and was on the respirator 24 hours a day. After 2 weeks my brain activity was stronger. My family was then told I would live but be in a vegetative state. They began taking me off the respirator for short periods and I was now able to close my eyes. I remember being given a pain test, it felt like a pizza cutter was rolled over my big toenail and I jerked my foot away. It appeared that I had sensation but the doctors highly doubted that I would walk again. My family was told I would have constant pneumonia and UTIs, but I have never had pneumonia or UTIs.

I was starting to stabilize, showed more signs of consciousness and was off the respirator more, so I was moved to the neurology ward on an acute care floor. Those early days were confusing for me. I couldn't move my body, but had full sensation. I was severely injured but hadn't had surgery, my artery had fixed itself. Until the day I saw my Family Doctor, I seriously had told myself that this was not real but seeing him made me crumble and acknowledge my truth. I cried so hard for days and wished to die. My mother told me to suck it up because I had kids to think of. There and then my goal was to be the mother that my kids needed.

No doctor thought I was cognitively intact; my mom could tell and some nurses too. I disliked my Neurologist and faked sleep when he was around, which the nurses noticed. They encouraged me to show him I was responsive, and the next day, I made it clear to him that I was awake and responsive. The following day I was tested. The test was pictures! I'm a calculus teacher and they had me look at pictures! They then believed my mom and started physiotherapy as well as putting in a tracheostomy tube and gastric tube. The first time I saw my limp face and body in a mirror at physiotherapy, I cried. I don't think of myself as vain but that was a real blow to my ego.

It had been a month since I'd seen my kids. Since I no longer had so many tubes, my family decided to let them come. Our daughter was so happy to see me. She didn't cry but I sure did. My stepson was almost 9 and had a new Gameboy that allowed him to be in his own world, I hurt for him so much! From 11-4 each day I got to be with Grace and my mom. Bill would come after work, stay for a while and then take Grace home while mom stayed until 7. I was still upset but there was no doubt in my mind that I would recover and have another child. I had pictures on the walls of the kids. There was one picture of me from before the stroke on the wall behind my bedhead. Before I went to sleep, I tried to tilt my head back and look at that picture.

Around 2 months after my stroke I started to regain neck movement. At 3 months, my laugh and cry noises returned. I still had double vision, the muscles around my left eye were weak so that eye drifted towards my nose. The circulation in my feet was still concerning me and having a limp expressionless face was hard for me to take. Around then I was told I was ready to go to the physical rehabilitation hospital.

Things were progressing and I had just learned to use the letterboard. I was told to spell out how I felt which was "FUCK!" I felt it summed up my feelings well. My mom giggled. I was excited to go to rehab, but also nervous because it meant a new environment, more hopes and fears. Since I was a young woman with young children and couldn't speak, I was given a private room across from the nurses' station. When I was checked in, I was told I would get physical therapy (PT), occupational therapy (OT), speech and language therapy (SLP) and the nurses would work on potty training with me. The first time my OT visited my room, she started fitting me for my new wheelchair. That night I cried so hard, I was overwhelmed and nervous about my future!

Each morning, I spent 50 minutes at each therapy, then the afternoons went for walks with Grace and my mom. In PT we worked on sitting and during OT sessions I learned to drive an electric wheelchair with my head movements. During my SLP appointments they quickly ran out of things to do with me as speaking was my greatest weakness. When Bill finished work each day, he would come and spend time with us. He would take Grace to have supper. Mom stayed with me until about 8 each day. There was no pulling her away from me; she stayed by my side for the next 17 years.

I wish I could say that rehab solved all my issues, but it didn't. I was there for 7 months; maybe more time would have helped, but progress slowed. In 2005 the team informed me that they believed that any improvement would only happen in the first year. Rehab nurses had helped me with my bladder and bowels, my tracheostomy was removed, and I learned to use the head array for the electric wheelchair. I was shaken that I didn't improve physically. I had grown up as a dancer from the age of 4. In high school and university I played sports. Who was I if I was no longer that person? Bill insisted that I come back to the family home. Bill has a disabled sister, so he grew up with disability and was not afraid of my many challenges.

I was so happy to be going home. It was a week before Christmas and two weeks before Grace's 2nd Birthday. I was excited but boy did I cry! I was scared, apprehensive and overwhelmed and poor William, my stepson, saw it all. It is sad to think of young children dealing with these emotions, but their presence really helped to distract me from my reality. My mother stayed with Grace and me while Bill was at work, then Bill stayed with us at night. My mother made everything possible and basically raised my child. When William was 11, he came to live with us full-time. Thanks to my mother and mother-in-law, that transition went well.

The first 5 years at home and being in a new body was hard for me. I clung to Bill. I went to sleep each night fearing I would die in my sleep, rarely left the house and feared my own shadow. How do you learn to trust your body again? I started hating myself for acting like a victim. I was nothing like the person I once was. I wanted my old self back, but I was stuck.

I spent 7 years not being able to talk to my children, 7 years of not being able to hug and kiss them. I got to be present in their lives and that had to be enough. In the early days, Grace would pretend to use the letterboard with me. She was never shy or scared with me, but William was a different story. William knew me pre-stroke, so this was hard on him and he was quiet around me. I had started venturing out more and went with the family to a basketball tournament. Some gyms were accessible, and some weren't, so I sat in the van for a few games. I was going to swimming classes, skating classes and basketball games but I still wasn't talking.

At this point, I started to live in a fantasy world and I stopped pushing myself to improve. Bill started to get frustrated that I wasn't looking for a better way to communicate. Bill finally got through to me and I reached out for help. I got a computer that I controlled with my head movements. It let me talk without needing an interpreter and I now had access to the internet which meant I could talk to more people! So much is said about how bad the internet is, but I just see joy. Since I no longer clung to Bill, he was able to get out of the house more and spend time with friends.

When I got my computer, Grace was 9 and William was 16. I chose to have a British accent when I spoke. Grace thought I was way too bossy now and was frustrated that she couldn't speak for me anymore. William was now a sullen teenager. When he was 14 his mother passed away and I will forever wish that I could have done more for him at that time.

I didn't eat by mouth for 10 years. I liked the taste of food when I ate it, but I never had cravings for things. When I was fully conscious in acute care for the first time, I did have a huge craving for kiwi and watermelon, I wanted water in my mouth so badly! Quickly, I learned to let that desire go. I failed the barium swallow test twice and learned that water is the hardest thing to swallow. When I came home from rehab, I started eating mashed potatoes. I found eating made my jaw sore, so I stopped eating by mouth and eating became just a source of fuel for my body. Being strictly tube fed didn't bother me. After 10 years my opinion changed; I wanted to try eating by mouth again. One day I said to myself "screw it, if I die, I die". I started sucking on chocolate, then Bill bought a Vitamix and away we went. I can eat cut up soft foods because my chewing is weak. I dislike the texture of pureed foods so my vegetable intake is poor. I tube feed for breakfast and then eat my lunch and supper by mouth. I keep one meal tube feed to keep up my fluids because I don't feel that my intake of fluids by mouth is adequate.

The electric wheelchair with the head array collected a lot of dust. When I came home from rehab, I was in a house with a toddler and did not want to try out my new wheelchair. When I hit a bump outside, the controls got misaligned. The chair was cumbersome, it didn't fit into my van well. I returned the chair to my province's health authority. In 2019, I tried a chin-controlled chair simply because I was awed by the actor Bryan Cranston in a movie.

In the fall of 2010, William started high school and Grace started grade 1. School was social time for Will; schoolwork was not his favorite thing. He stuck with it and got his diploma in 2014. Grace always loved school and I tried very hard to be an involved parent. One day my cousin had Grace with her and her daughter Emma. Grace was 7, Emma was 4. Emma asked Grace what it was like to have me as a mom. Grace said that I was like all moms, but I just couldn't walk or talk. My cousin was very excited to tell me that story.

By 2017 I'd had a computer for 4 years and had not yet searched 'Brainstem Stroke' - that's how deep my disregard for reality was. These are old stats, but they shook me; 1% of strokes are in the brainstem and in 90% of those cases the patient dies. No wonder the doctors kept telling my family that I would most likely die. There are people that are fully "Locked-In", with no movement at all, and I had the nerve to feel sorry for myself! My outlook on my life changed that day.

In 2018, Grace was starting high school and Will had moved to another city. I knew that I needed to start thinking about my future. In April of that year, there was a terrible hockey team bus crash. 16 people died and 14 were left injured. A call went out for trauma counselors, and I found my future. I had a working brain and a wealth of experience with trauma.

I found an online university and got started. I knew painfully little about how computers worked. I needed to take four prerequisite classes before I could apply for the master's program in counseling. I had to admit I had physical deficits and that I read slower. I went through the disability office and got an accommodation for added time on exams.

A month after I started my second course, COVID hit. Life was turning upside down, but I still had five more months to finish my course. I wasn't fazed by COVID; my life is a continuous lock down. I took the last two classes, enjoyed them and prepared to apply for the counseling program.

In 2019, I read an article about a group in San Francisco that was changing brain signals into spoken words. My first thought was that this tool could really help me be a counselor. I moved on with my courses, but the brain signal study was in the back of my mind. In 2021, my brother sent me a link to a story about a guy that had a brainstem stroke who was participating in that study I had read about. Later that day, someone in my online support group posted a NYT article about the same guy. I thought, "why not me too"! I googled Doctor Edward Chang and wrote him in an email that I wanted to volunteer.

For years, Bill had tried to get me to join studies. In my eyes, being in a study meant moving away from my children. It was now the summer before Grace entered grade 12. I felt it was time for mom to become Ann again.

I quickly heard back from the study coordinator. We set up our initial zoom meeting where Bill and I met with the coordinator. We introduced ourselves, talked about the study and the guidelines for test subjects then asked if we had questions. Here comes the road bump… Bill said "We're Canadian, is that an issue"?

She told us if we were willing to relocate to the San Francisco Bay Area, it was a go. I was determined for this to become reality so I put my schooling on hold. It was made clear that this study would not improve my life, but it might help future generations. I was a teacher, and teachers always want to help others.

I had spent a year working with the coordinator and the doctors. Where to live, how often we'd go back to Canada and getting FDA approval. This all took place in 2021/2022 during COVID and border issues were involved.

I had applied to a local charity to help us buy a new van. We were approved for help getting an accessible van to get me there. After several letdowns, we found a caregiver willing to work with me. The plan was for Bill to stay in the Bay Area for 3 weeks then fly back home for 3 weeks. While he was home, the caregiver flew down to stay with me.

We drove into San Francisco to get formal approval for the study. We met the study coordinator, Margaret, who we had been working with for over a year. Next, we met the doctors for a general health and physical condition check. The major item was an MRI. I was also having a fMRI and a contrast MRI. I spent 3 hours in the MRI tube, it makes the loudest noise. I was so happy to get out of that tube and go home to bed.

The following Sunday I met Dr. Chang. He was unlike any Neurologist or Neurosurgeon I'd met before. He was 35-40 and had a personality. In my experience these professionals are often old and difficult to have a conversation with. The first thing he said was that I had a beautiful brain. I think I fell in love with him right then! I wasn't scared about the surgery, I was excited.

Before I had left Regina, I had shaved my head for my surgery, and sent everyone messages that I loved them. I remember focusing on my breathing and trying to relax. The surgery was about 7 hours and went very well. I woke up in the recovery room to Bill and a lot of pain. Staples in the head and antibiotics that made me nauseous. After surgery, I spent four more days in the hospital. Bill stayed with me at nights and slept on a pull-out chair. Bill is 6'4".

One day Dr. Chang and the team came and plugged me in. They ran tests to make sure everything was running correctly. I started to feel better. When Dr. Chang talks, his voice is comforting; a world-renowned Neurosurgeon talking to me like he was my neighbor, I felt so safe!

Having something sticking out of your head is a very odd feeling and staples and stitches in your scalp are painful. Dr. Chang checked on me often in the following two weeks, the pain was getting better but the nausea stayed. It felt so odd when the cap was twisted off the port that was screwed to my skull. Dr. Chang said that I was the first human to have this array and the only cap they had was primate proof! A few weeks after the surgery I had half of my staples removed. Mainly they did not hurt to remove, but the ones behind the ear and by the temple were sensitive. On day ten after the surgery, we started the exciting journey of data collection.

During the first 8 weeks, we met five days a week, four hours each day. When the team wanted to try new things we met on weekends also. My mouth needed to be woken up after not being used for all those years. My tongue felt like a dead fish, there was so much extra saliva being produced so I coughed a lot the first week or two. It blew my mind that my brain remembered how to move my mouth to form words. I felt my enunciation was not good enough, looked up speech therapy on YouTube then practiced mouth movements for each letter. Somehow my brain took in that information and made that information useful. Having been an athlete and a coach, I noticed that the same thing happens when you train for sports. I was in awe of the brain's power and loved the feedback we were getting. I was volunteering for this study so the science could be pushed forward, but also found I loved helping researchers see what the brain could do, I got to be a teacher again!

The first few weeks we collected a lot of data where I would mouth the NATO alphabet and everyday phrases. The first time we tested NATO, the model algorithm got 70%. The researchers were excited. Over the next couple of weeks, we climbed to 80%, 90% and even 100%. Researchers were cheering. I was told this was a world first. I just couldn't believe how easy it was, it was the computer and researchers that did all the work.

Next, attention was directed toward trying to translate 50 everyday phrases. The model algorithm got the entire phrases correct except for 2-4 words. Accuracy improved each day until one day we got to 97%. The researchers had converted brain signals to text.

The next step was to make my newly made voice say that text. I had brought a videotape of me speaking at our wedding twenty years ago. The researchers used that video to make a synthetic voice with attributes of my voice from that recording. I don't understand how this researcher streamed the voice and text together. Many times I was in awe of the researchers.

They were also introducing the avatar at the same time. The team had me pick out an avatar to represent myself. I chose one that was young and pretty. The fact that they got the avatar's mouth movements to go at the same time as text and synthesis was wonderful; again, I was in awe. They also had me make facial expressions and the avatar would show those expressions.

I need to emphasize how important it is for a person to have a purpose, to feel that they're contributing to society. I loved feeling useful again. The team came to me each day and it made me feel like I had something special to offer. They showed me so much respect and constantly asked for my input. They treated me like a person and weren't afraid of me.

In mid-November 2022 we returned to Canada. We completed many demonstration videos before I left. I relaxed and spent time with my family while the team wrote a 49-page paper. When we returned in January, everything still worked well. We spent January refining the avatar and the research team finished writing the paper which was submitted to the journal, Nature.

I didn't fully understand how huge our progress was. Some days Dr. Chang would come by and have a sly smile, you could tell he was pleased when he watched our decoding. When peer reviews came back, they were mostly positive but one thought that I was actually speaking aloud; I took that as a compliment. After the work was done to satisfy the peer reviewers the article was accepted by Nature.

All winter we did new tasks. In the spring, UCSF's media department got involved, created a video and wrote an article. Now we waited for the Nature article to come out. It was time to head back to Canada, catch up on life at home and sort out some marital issues with Bill.

The following August, I spoke with a reporter from the New York Times and a photographer came to my house. I now understood how big this was. At the same time my scalp started to recede from the post on my head. When the paper was published in Nature, the NYT article came out and it was on the front page! There was my 15 minutes of fame and it was worldwide.

When I returned, we were doing new tasks. There were some new researchers to get to know. I was still struggling with our marital issues, but didn't dwell on them. In October I developed an infection around the port on my head. I had known from the beginning that this was a possibility but hearing Dr. Chang say that the implant might have to be removed was a blow. Meanwhile, the team was asked to present at the White House. I was told President Biden watched the video. There were many rounds of antibiotics, but the infection never resolved. On Jan. 25, 2024, my implant was removed.

This time there were no staples; plastic surgeon Dr. Hoffman stitched me up. I was on antibiotics for eight weeks, was given the all clear and no infection remained. The study continues but it was time for our story in the study to end. I got to feel that I had a purpose again, I truly felt I had contributed.

It is June 12th, 2024, and I'm not dead yet! This journey started almost 20 years ago, I'm now almost 50 and I've learned a lot along the way. Happiness is never guaranteed, it's a choice you make every day. Every person alive has struggles and they're doing their best. Everyone needs to feel they have value and that they can contribute to the world in some way. We as humans are so hard on ourselves, I know I was. I had no idea this could even happen to a person, and I think I've made the best out of the cards I was dealt.

Editor's note: Please see chapter 3 for details about the brain-computer-interface research that Ann participated in with Dr. David Moses and the team at the Chang Lab at UCSF.

8   The Second Life of Mario Bros

Bénédicte Jullien

I feel a bit like Mario and having multiple lives! Same decor, same surroundings, but a very different life.

I am an ordinary citizen like you. I come from Liège, Belgium. I studied as a special education teacher and worked in various fields such as people with mental disabilities, prisons, homeless people. But what I did the most was work with children and young people.

My main passion is and remains travel. With Alexandre, my boyfriend at the time and future husband, we lived in Ireland for two years, did a ski season in France and travelled around Latin America for a year. I also moved around a lot solo before but for shorter stays. In short, travel is very important to me. Otherwise, I was a good living person who liked to eat and drink and go out too. In summary, I loved life and that is surely what will save me. But of course, before the stroke, as newlyweds with young children, we were calmer. But this stroke will certainly have taught me to enjoy life, which I was already doing, but here and now, it is irresponsible to wait. Because we don't know what tomorrow will bring. If I had been told, for example, that from November 13, 2016, I would no longer set foot in any of the rooms in the house and that I would leave it and my loved ones, I would not have believed it.

November 12, 2016

I called the doctor on November 10, 2016, two days before. It's not my style to call him. In six and a half years, it's quite simple, at work, I have been absent twice. Once, for a day without a certificate and the second time for a week because I had sprained my foot. In short, as far as I remember, I never asked him for a certificate. I'm not very complaining about my health, even though I have a great need to understand what's going on.

I had to feel this was important. For two days I had white holes, as I call them. These were significant vision problems. Like a white veil falling before the eyes. What is very scary is driving with your children on board. It's very simple, I stopped several times on the way. You are afraid of having an accident or losing control of your vehicle.

DOI: 10.4324/9781003464181-8

Doctor's diagnosis, I'm a little tired and I'm lacking iron. He tells me to call him on Monday if things don't get better. But Monday will be too late. I blame him. Not for diagnosis because he did manual tests to check that I wasn't having a stroke. Certainly, the tests were not alarming but it was in preparation. But I blame him for the fact that he doesn't see me often, that should have alerted him to my symptoms. It seems to me that prescribing an MRI in my case would not have been a luxury for someone who is not used to complaining or consulting. But it is obvious to me that he is a bad doctor. Taking 5 to 10 minutes per patient (which he practices), it is obvious that errors must exist.

On the morning of November 12, I sent a first text message to Alexandre, my husband. I'm hungry but I don't feel the strength to go down. I'm in my room on the second floor of the house. Very kindly, he goes upstairs with the children and a plate. I still remember it was homemade cake with a cup of milk. He comes back down with the children and advises me to rest.

I can barely eat. The food I hoped would be beneficial doesn't do anything for me. I'm still too weak to go down. I send a second text saying I'm not feeling well. This too is rare. In eleven years of dating, I wonder if this has ever happened. Alex, my husband is coming up. He no longer understands what I'm saying. But I remember concentrating on saying the word toilet. I have the strange feeling that the words are coming out of my mouth distorted. I never tell myself or realize that I am having a stroke, it is not possible. Fortunately, Alex understood. I had read about what a stroke was, but I didn't remember it. I was convinced that this only happens to others and when I'm older. So I had time before having to find out. I was very naive.

I don't know by what miracle, but he understands that I have to go to the bathroom. He carries me down the stairs, like a princess. The toilets are one floor down, like the children's bedroom. At that moment, I was very far from imagining that I would leave this room forever. My body has already given up on me. And barely down, I'm incontinent. My children saw it all. I'm lying on the ground; I feel like I'm getting on top of myself. But I don't care. My son, 4 years old at the time, brings me his cushion, because I am lying on the floor. My daughter, almost two years old, cries, alone, in front of my empty bed. Very quickly, Alex will call the neighbour for help. Later, my son will ask his father why he was yelling at me. Was he angry? He kept me awake. Thanks to him, I won't have a coma.

Help is arriving. We wait in the ambulance parked in front of the house, I will never understand why. I remember lying on a stretcher and laughing inside. I imagined the neighbours at their door or window. We lived at that time in the countryside, in a dead-end street. Suffice to say that the entertainment is rare. As you can imagine, I was far from thinking that it was serious. For me, as I felt good, I was going to go home in the evening.

I transform into LiS. I had made my life, 2 young children and a charming husband, great trips, lots of outings. In short, I took advantage of it. I was certain that nothing could happen to me except an accident, illness or death. Certainly not, being disabled, completely paralyzed with a tube down your throat!

I didn't know about locked in syndrome. Unlike those around me, I understood late what I had. Well, without words, it is difficult to ask questions, to ask for details. Especially since the medical world was unknown to me until then. I have obviously already gone to visit someone in the hospital, but without paying attention to the many noises. Indeed, the hospital (intensive care) is full of different noises, unknown to me. Indeed, there are a lot of beeps in every corner, slamming doors. Sometimes, even if it's rare, the silence is total, without the noise of cars, as if death were overtaking you. When you hear people running; you tell yourself it's not good and pray it doesn't happen in your room. When you have visitors, people speak softly, as if you were dead. In short, the impression is persistent of death lurking.

After

One of the first thoughts I had when I became disabled was that from now on, having pain would be my daily life.

Indeed, without actions or words, you can only endure what is happening.

Suffering when the nurse catches your hand while turning you in bed; suffer when you turn, you encounter a pillow which prevents you from breathing freely, suffer when the strap of the lift cuts into your thigh because it is poorly worn; suffer when your pelvis is poorly positioned… The examples are countless. I thought I would never be comfortable in my body again, without pain, like an able-bodied person can be.

But fortunately, the body gets used to it.

When I returned home, after a year and a half in hospital, I learned unpleasantly about non- verbal language, a language without words, gestures, or any alternative means of communication.

Why unpleasant?

Without gestures or words, you must make yourself understood. There remains the movement of your eyes.

It's not much. Many people will not understand this language. You can explain to them that you have to follow your gaze, that it gives the direction of what you want to talk about, instead of pointing, they will not understand.

Therefore, no communication will be possible. Added to this are uncontrollable emotions.

Between your incomprehensible crying and the non-verbal communication which is very easily interpreted in a negative way, the majority of caregivers take you for a mean person and there is nothing you can do about it. In my city, I am on the red list of most nurses. Patient too difficult, with too severe a handicap compared to the renumeration.

Imagine yourself in your bed, lying down. Without moving or speaking, make your interlocutor understand that your pelvis is in the wrong position.

With experience, the nurse knows that she must only ask questions with a yes or no answer, and that a question must also be broken down to get a more precise answer. For example, are you in pain? To know where, you have to break down the body: above? Yes or no? Between? Yes or no? Down? Yes or no? Then, when you know the area, you have to break down this area. OK, it's at the top, we'll find where. Head? Yes or no? Shoulders? Yes or no, etc.

During this very long time, you suffer and in silence please! In silence, because if you express your pain, your interlocutor will be paralyzed by your very strong and incomprehensible emotion and will become incapable of thinking, immobilized by fear. And as a result, you will endure the pain even longer. So, the experience taught me to endure without even showing it on my face.

I remember one time when my helper had put the lift strap on very badly. Once in the air, I cried out in pain. At the same time, she raised the bed for her back. My cry coming at the same time, she concluded that I didn't want her to get back into bed and began to explain to me why it was important. She spoke while leaving me in the air and I screamed even more!

A prerequisite for this communication is kindness, because it is easier to interpret than to understand what the other really means and even more so when their reality is different.

For example, I often ask that the lift cover be centred; that to sleep, my arms are extended; that my joystick or my computer is placed to the nearest centimeter and these are just a few examples. One can easily conclude that I am demanding. In fact, the side strap hurts me; the weight of the duvet is too great to allow me to lift it to be able to extend my arm which if it remains bent will hurt me and the computer (or the joystick) poorly placed a few millimeters is unusable due to my almost non-existent mobility.

So, without always understanding why, you have to agree to do things. Fortunately for my nurses, these benchmarks are always the same.

Non-verbal communication requires many other rules. For the interlocutor as well as for me. For example, for me, I must observe every gesture of my interlocutor. Indeed, if I want to be able to communicate information about something, I have to talk about it at the precise moment when the person acts on this thing and it depends on the second.

Example, I want to say that today, I would like my black hair clip. If I say it before or after she does my hair, even if I look in the direction of the hair clip, she won't understand me. It is essential to contextualize the topic of conversation by choosing exactly the moment to intervene.

So, between constant observation, being in pain or cold in silence and trying to stay calm to be able to get a message across, non-verbal communication is exhausting. And all this while trying to control these uncontrollable emotions.

And the interlocutor is not left out. He must constantly be on the lookout for the slightest sign that perhaps constitutes an attempt at communication. If he has slept poorly or is ill, his observation will be impaired and communication will be much more difficult. And with my uncontrollable emotions,

I could burst into tears because this difficulty will be too much. So my poor interlocutor, in addition to being sick, may have to manage a crisis.

No matter how much you explain that it is non-verbal communication that is like that, that it is no one's fault, the person will be frustrated and will spread the word that you are an impossible patient to take care of. So you will then have difficulty finding a nurse who has not been influenced by what he says.

Fortunately, there are some nurses who understand this language. According to specialists in non-verbal communication, you must have the same type of education to have the same codes.

This is indeed a good start. Unfortunately, this is not enough. As I said above, you need kindness and patience.

I too learned patience and letting go very early on. Indeed, when you want to say something, it takes so long that you have to learn patience. Example, you are poorly dressed, it hurts you.

You will need time to write it and once it is finally finished, just as you were about to say the sentence, your young child asks for his dad to go to the toilet. So you suffer in silence.

Another example, you see that a domestic accident is going to occur. By the time you write to alert, the accident will have occurred! So you learn to observe by letting go. It's just horrible but you have no choice. So, I learned to anticipate potential dangers without making it a phobia either.

One of my other big frustrations at the beginning was not being able to say anything the first fifteen minutes after waking up. Indeed, my computer takes a long time to turn on. Afterwards, you need time to write this first sentence.

The first years are truly hell. We've already talked about non-verbal communication and the difficulty of not being able to say anything when you wake up. But that's only a few things. Added to this is the invasion of new emotions which make me feel guilty, the way people look at me and their habit of speaking about me in the third person when I am present, accepting that they speak to me as if they were a child or that they caress my head like an animal, the kisses or cuddles that my loved ones no longer give, new pains, the ban on drinking or eating, the obligation to defecate in a diaper, waiting for all my primary needs, not being able to satisfy any of my desires, stay in bed continuously because the house is not suitable, be a burden for the people who take care of me and accept comments in silence… The list is of course not exhaustive.

I am relatively lucky to be in Belgium. I have access to speech therapy and physiotherapy. I have food to eat every day and financial aid for adapted equipment. Compared to many countries, I am lucky. But unfortunately, all this just allows me to breathe and keeps me healthy, but nothing more.

When I returned home, the state offered me the necessary adaptations at home, except that my house was unadaptable.

On several floors, only the narrow living room was accessible to me. So in this room, there was now my double bed with my husband. In the rest of the room, my wardrobe, my chair, a lift, a dining table and it was in this small space that the four of us lived. Which meant that I had no room to move. So, I lived 24 hours a day in my bed. One more difficulty. Fortunately for us, we are fighters. We organized a fundraiser which allowed us to build a suitable house.

But that is not the only difficulty. At the hospital, as you could call a nurse whenever you wanted, I was taught continence. But back home, there is no one to help you go to the toilet and so the state offers you diapers free of charge! So, today and for 6 years, I am stagnating every day in my stools or my urine!

The immense difficulty I encounter is not having anyone to satisfy my primary needs, and therefore even less any desire. Eating or drinking when I need to, going to the bathroom, taking a nap, taking a shower, putting on a sweater, etc., are needs that I cannot satisfy at the moment. Simple desires like going for a walk, gardening or go buy a treat are completely inaccessible to me.

So, I think that LiS people who continue to survive this hell of the early years are strong, fighting people. That if the population knew a quarter of what we went through, they absolutely would not believe it.

My Secret to Keeping Going

My children and projects.

It all started with a fund-raising campaign to create an adapted house, because my house at the time was too small to be able to live there in a chair. So we appealed for donations. This fund- raising enabled us to build a house entirely adapted to my needs.

Then, from this fundraiser, a Facebook page was created where I explain what it means to be disabled to the 4,000 people who read me.

I love travelling. But adapted accommodation is rare. So, with my husband, in 2021, we created a gîte adapted to my needs. We also rent it out.

Given the deplorable situation for people with severe disabilities in Belgium, to try and change things, a few friends and I have set up the Belgian association of locked in syndrome (BALIS). The association is very young, but very active nonetheless.

And After Several Years?

Tranquillity is no longer part of my life. However, fortunately, I am getting used to some things. I know the intensity of emotions, the first quarter of an hour of the day is a habit, I have resigned myself to the way people look…

After long years of waiting (7!), I finally had access to a budget to satisfy my basic needs. Basically, it is no longer my loved ones who have to take care of me but professionals. They come at several key moments of the day. But I always have to wait for the agreed time to eat, drink, stop stagnating in my excrement... So, my needs are always postposed. And when it comes to desire, I can go for a walk in the neighbourhood, but on the street, because the sidewalks are unsuitable and therefore impassable in 80% of cases. This also makes me feel like I live in an underdeveloped country.

The lack of affection or the inability to satisfy desires remain very difficult things to live with. For that, Belgian social security, which means that I do not have a companion, does not make my life easier! This is no longer the case in many countries. So, I hope that my situation will change. In any case, I'm fighting for this because I don't accept that we can live in these conditions. It's bordering on inhumane!

9 Communication Without Speech

Bex Kemp

Frustrating. That is how I would best describe locked-in syndrome.

I was a happy thirty-two-year old living in Cheltenham, UK, with my friend and cat.

I was a communication manager for an environmental organisation, volunteered at the local animal shelter and also volunteered walking dogs for the elderly and people who couldn't.

I loved to swim and did some charity swims for diabetes as my best friend has type one. I enjoyed badminton with my family and I loved to horse ride. Playing piano was another hobby of mine.

I may as well have had a bed in my kitchen as that is where I spent most of my free time as I loved to cook. Whilst I was in the Intensive Care Unit (ICU) mum used to bring me in things to smell to allow me to still enjoy smells at least. I would try to guess what it was and I must say I was quite good as my sense of smell is intact.

I also played violin for The Cheltenham Philharmonic Orchestra. My family really enjoyed watching me performing at various venues around Cheltenham.

I had not long returned from the USA as I used to travel a lot for my work when my devastating brainstem stroke happened. It was the 30th of November, 2019, and I was just getting ready to meet my family; it really just goes to show that anything can happen to anyone without a warning. I remember the day, like it was yesterday, but I won't go into the details except that I knew something was up, when my eyes locked to the right. My parents took me to the local hospital, as advised by the Paramedics, (even though they did not have a Stroke unit) - the ambulance service said they were so busy they could not say how long it would take for an ambulance to arrive or take me to hospital.

At hospital, my friend said he thought I was having a stroke but the doctors would not listen and said I was too young. I was transferred from the first hospital to the second hospital by ambulance, but there was no urgency as the ambulance crew didn't use either the siren or the blue lights and stopped at all the traffic lights.

DOI: 10.4324/9781003464181-9

When I got to the second hospital (that actually had a Stroke unit), they said they were unsure if I had suffered a Stroke. I didn't really understand what was going on.

I can't really recall what happened after being transferred to the second hospital but my mum has told me that at one stage they did a swallow test with some water and I coughed when trying to drink the water. At some point I was moved to a side ward. Later that evening, my mum said I really deteriorated and she demanded the doctors come and look at me again. It was after this that I was admitted to the intensive care unit (ICU).

I had had several CT scans, one with higher contrast, but my family were initially told they didn't show a clot. An MRI scan was done and it was later confirmed that I had suffered a stroke. By that time, it was too late to give me the clot busting drug.

I remember I had a lot of vivid dreams in the early days, and I can still remember them nearly five years on. I also have some very strong memories of around the hospital. I think even though it took a long time for the stroke to be picked up, it was recognised early on in ICU that I was fully cognitive.

When I left ICU and went onto the Stroke ward, a lovely Charity called "Special Effect" supported me, providing an Eye gaze tablet, with Grid three software, so I could access emails, Facebook, WhatsApp and a web browser.

This support was handed over to the NHS' Electronic Assistive Technology department (EAT), in Bristol, and they have spent lots of time fine tuning my tablet and means of typing on a virtual keyboard. This tablet has two cameras attached to it, which are calibrated to my eyes, enabling me to type text using just my eyes. The NHS's Augmentative and Alternative Communication department (AAC) enabled me to control my TV, Amazon, Netflix, YouTube and other programmes, plus turn my bedside lamp on and off, using a head button attached to both my wheelchair and my bed. I can also request help from ward staff using this button. They have, in the last two weeks, added my cooling fan speed, on and off and oscillation, to my head button, which is another bit of control that is important to me as my room can get very hot.

My Great Aunt bought an electric wheelchair, for her to possibly use, after upcoming surgery, but she allowed me to use it until she needs it. It has a Standing facility, and this helps with my bowel activity, as I use it to stand every day.

I was categorised as Nil by mouth (NBM) but for a short time was receiving liquidised food, orally, from the unit I am currently at. The Speech & Language (SLT) lady left and that input stopped. My parents, for three years or so, were increasing my oral intake, with a wide variety of liquidised food. I loved my food so my mum used to include me in most of the meals they were having, even takeaways, and I got to the point that I was receiving 75% of my daily nutrition, orally. However, I caught flu, which led to a chest infection and pneumonia. I was not told but, apparently, on three separate occasions, two of the doctors and the Consultant disclosed to mum and dad that I was not responding to the very powerful antibiotic I was on and that they didn't think I was going to pull through. After a three-week spell in the Respiratory Ward, a massive dose of steroids, three additional antibiotics, and a huge input from the Respiratory Physios two and three times per day, I pulled through, but it left me even more tired than I usually am and my oxygen readings had dropped from 98 to 94.

I have always wanted to better myself and keep myself occupied. Before I was in hospital with pneumonia, I was full of energy and did lots of therapies which I did enjoy and I was getting results from. I found that after I became very much compromised by being poorly, I had no energy and all therapies needed to stop as I was too tired to do them.

My therapies ranged from relaxing to hard work. I had reflexology and acupuncture which are both relaxing and I just enjoyed them as I did not have to do anything. I have physio, at my current residence, working on my neck strength and standing on the tilt table which is good for my neck strength and organs. I'm still receiving stretches provided where I live and that is great for keeping all my limbs supple. I also have a private physio once a week and we worked on a range of movements especially my neck. I also do hydrotherapy. I was an avid swimmer and I swam a lot; the water is very much where I feel most comfortable. I work to music and it's good for the body as you can do exercises in water that you just cannot do on land. Hydro is very tough but I get a lot out of it and I work extremely hard. My therapist is really good and very positive. My mum is in the pool with us to enable the Hydrotherapist to do more exercises. He is always trying different positions and gadgets. I also do Hippotherapy which even though it has hippo in the title has nothing to do with hippos, but we managed to fool a few carers into thinking it did, which kept me amused! Anyway, it is actually riding a horse; in my case, I ride a mechanical horse which walks, trots, canters, gallops and feels just like a real horse. I know because I was a great horse rider. I used to do dressage and jumping. I spent a lot of time with horses. I can sit on a mechanical horse nearly unaided. Muscle memory is a powerful thing. I'm a quadriplegic so it is a big deal. The Hippotherapist believes that I will be able to ride a real horse at some point in the not too distant future.

I also have Neurological Music Therapy. In music I vocalise as much as possible whilst the therapist sings and plays either the keyboard or the acoustic guitar. I am unable to form actual words but I try to be as vocal as I can. I have a bit of movement in the tip of my right middle finger so we use an Orba device to exercise my finger to see if it can be functional. I have not given up on regaining sufficient finger control, or utilising another part of my body, to allow me to control my electric wheelchair.

I've been told I have a severe case of Locked-in Syndrome (LiS) so need a high level of support.

I have always been close to my family but LiS has definitely brought us together. I discuss with my parents things I never thought I would. My brother has been amazing and I see him often. He takes me out and enables me to see my friends and, if possible, I am even closer to him than I was before. We have the same group of friends which helped.

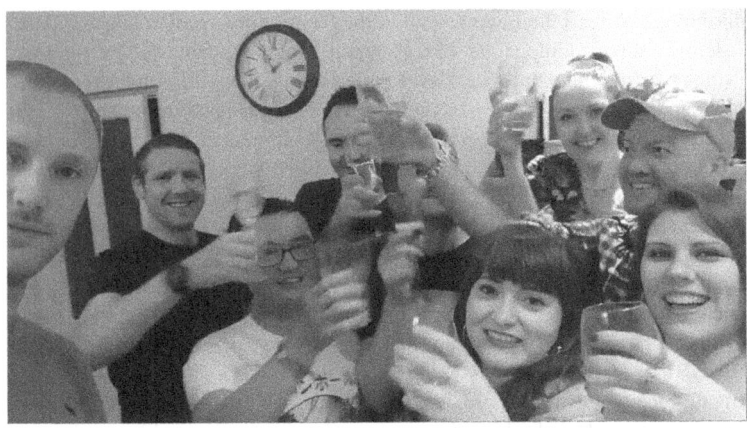

Figure 9.1 My friends and I enjoying one of our many evenings together. Bex is bottom right.

I feel that I am not as close to my friends because even though they try to include me in events there are only certain things they can include me in. I also have issues with visiting their houses as obviously they are built for able people. Of course, I don't blame anyone as I would not expect anyone to alter their houses just for me. I would not even expect my parents to alter their place for me. I'm not the people who have to live there.

One of the most frustrating things is communicating with staff/people who won't use my spelling board and just ask "Closed" questions, so I am prevented from saying what I want to. When being put to bed, or readied for sleep, it is possible, just asking closed questions, to position my "V" pillow correctly. I have a neck pillow that helps stop my neck muscles pulling my head to my left and this has to be in a certain position to enable me to comfortably watch TV plus allow me to turn to access my Eye Gaze tablet for emailing, WhatsApping, and Facebook, etc. I have a sausage pillow, between the bottom of my bed and the soles of my feet, to help stop "Foot Drop." Sometimes I need two pillows if I am positioned higher up in my bed. This "Sleep system" is something that has been developed over years, and I like to have a staff member who is familiar with it all because my bed comfort is important as I can't move a single muscle myself.

It's also difficult when I know what I want to say, and say it in a brief form, but folk don't get the exact picture and guess wrong so I get frustrated and upset which then upsets them too.

I was assessed, about 4 years ago, and moved a wheelchair forward, but not having consistent control meant I could not always stop the chair which was dangerous.

When people are not looking at me continuously, they might not spot my eyelids fluttering to say "I want to spell" so I'm working hard to be able to make a sound, when required, to cause them to look at me at those times.

Not being able to breath in and out myself, means that when I need to cough, to clear my throat, or sniff to unblock my nose, it is maddening as I have to wait for my brain to detect the irritation and cough for me plus I have to ask people to clear my nose with a cotton bud.

My body thermostat was broken when I had my Stroke, so I feel the cold more which is annoying as I was a real outdoor girl. I had been a member of my local Scout Group, wandering around in winter with short sleeved tops on feeling like toast.

I, Bex, suggested that my Mum, Dad and brother Richard might want to contribute to my chapter.

So, Mum and Dad Wrote:

After Bex's stroke, she spent around three weeks in ICU, before moving onto a Stroke ward. We spent every one of those days with Bex, from after the doctors did their morning rounds to around 22.00 hrs. The hospital allowed us to sleep in a visitors' bedroom, which avoided us travelling to and from home every day.

She had such little control over her neck that she spent the early weeks laying in her bed and looking up at the ceiling. Mum bought her a small projector that shone a moving pattern on the ceiling, to break up her boredom.

The SLT suggested that, as Bex could not now speak, we consider a "Spelling/Alphabet" board to help us communicate with her. Mum was horrified at the thought of this as, in the very early days, we had hoped that movement and speech might return. You read that Stroke sufferers can recover many of their losses and this is what we had hoped for Bex. Eventually we gave it a try and bought a whiteboard and pen, to write down what she was going to say. It very quickly became apparent that Bex had retained her cognition, and sarcastic sense of humour, when the first phrase she spelt out, to dad, was "You are a nob" which was when we realised, "she was still all there." We have that board, at home, with her phrase written on it and will never forget the many Carers and staff that came to look at it, not believing what she had written. She looks up for "No," and down for "Yes," and flutters her eye-lids when she wants to spell.

This spelling system became something that we found we needed to make folk aware of as not many staff had seen it or could use it. It was a battle then and still continues to require us to constantly monitor it to enable Bex to be able to spell, to ask/reply to questions, and to tell people of any issues she has. Most staff just guessed questions and we produced a list of the common questions, but imagine trying to tell a person who could not use the board, "I have a hair in my right eye?"

We struggled in ICU and both of the next two rehab units Bex found herself in. Managers would say, "It's not the first language of the Carer, they may be dyslexic, they lack confidence." We still have nurses, and some Carers, where Bex is currently a resident, who prefer to guess or go and get another staff member who can spell with Bex.

Both BBC local radio and TV stations interviewed us all, and produced two very good articles on the spelling issue but both BBC National TV, and radio stations have ignored our contact emails to support a national campaign.

We discovered a great National charity, called "Remap" who find non-standard solutions for issues around communication and physical challenges for all sorts of conditions. When Bex was having her Neurological Music Therapy (NMT), they helped develop a piece of equipment that attached to Bex's wheelchair so the tiny movement, in one of her fingers, could be communicated to her in a way that she knew just how much she was moving it. This was particularly useful when she had a blanket over her. Bex used to spasm/cough/sneeze which, when in bed, caused her to move away from her head button and therefore unable to call staff for assistance. Remap devised a distance sensor that would trigger a bell to alert staff of this. Her neck control range has since improved so she has not needed it for several months now.

Their latest "gadget," which Bex is due to trial, will give feedback to Bex, and her NMT, about how hard she is pressing her "ORBA" https://www.andertons.co.uk/artiphon-orba-two. The ORBA allows Bex to make musical notes, with her single finger, but they are trying to determine if the strength of movement could be enough to, eventually, control her electric wheelchair.

Remap are happy to be approached.

Examples of their work: REMAP - Custom made equipment for disabled people. Main website: https://www.remapglos.org.uk

We applied for a Motability vehicle, as Bex has lots of hospital appointments and some private self-funded outside therapies, plus she loves to go to the local cinema and theatres to see shows. This was refused on the basis that "She is not entitled to a vehicle when in residential care which is funded by the NHS." We sold our own car, and bought a Wheelchair Accessible Vehicle (WAV) so we could take Bex wherever she wants to go. We have just appealed the decision so let's wait and see.

Bex has mentioned her previous oral feeding success, which was abruptly halted by her pneumonia and further affected by the recent Covid infection she had. Her SLT has said that she could consider "Eating for pleasure" but only after a full re-assessment of her lungs and swallow condition. We still hope that, as she gets stronger and begins to enjoy her food, that it may just become possible to re-try food for nutrition as well as pleasure. Bex still sees, and is in communication with, some of her previous work colleagues. Her employers were very supportive, and even though she is paralysed from the neck down and can't talk, they told her that if the technology existed, and Bex was able to use it, they would find a place for her in the organisation. She even received a visit from the Company's original CEO, who had travelled from Australia.

We still visit Bex six days per week for around five or six hours and she always has lots to say and important stuff to tell us. We know that as soon as she has recovered more of her strength, she will get back onto her therapies and we will see more improvements, and that she will ride an actual horse, with just a little support on each side from two helpers.

Mum Added:

Nobody can imagine how your life could change in just a day, that is what happened to our family. Our world was turned upside down and I can't imagine how Bex felt, not being able to tell us how she felt and must have been utterly devastating to her that she couldn't move one single muscle. How do you ever get over this, but Bex did.

I have found out so much about "My Little Girl." The strength and determination she has shown has blown my mind and her sense of humour has shone through. I think if Bex was any different, I'm sure I wouldn't have coped as well as I have. I'm so proud of how she has shown how strong she is, through every single day, to face the world with a smile on her face (well maybe not every day).

Dad Also Added:

Bex has always been a pedantic, and very precise, user of grammar, particularly with regards to her job as Communication Manager.

I quickly found that this was not about to change just because she had had a Stroke and the effort she puts into her communicating, using her spell board, is awesome.

It would be so simple for her to cut corners and accept peoples' near-enough guesses of her words as she constructs sentences, but she will only accept the precise spelling, despite some folks saying, "For goodness sake, Bex, I was nearly correct." Examples are "it's" will not be replaced by "it" and a singular will not be accepted, in place of the plural, if it does not fit grammatically.

Some of the words she uses to describe things often confound some of her Carers, who have never heard of them.

It continues to amaze me that, whilst dealing with all the things that come with her extensive Stroke disabilities, she maintains her standards, despite it requiring lots more effort.

It takes a lot longer to communicate, using a Spelling Board. I know it is easy to be impatient and we all suffer from that, so I do wonder how many other sufferers encounter folk who laugh when they nearly get it right, but the sufferer does not accept it.

I hope my previous sentence will encourage folk to consider what it's like, for the stroke victim, to want to say things the way they did before their Stroke, knowing that those who are communicating with them are showing impatience and don't get it.

Brother Richard's Words:

I am amazed how strong Bex remains despite what's happened. Throughout her ups and downs, which have consisted of mostly downs, she still remains as funny, bubbly and as thoughtful as ever. Despite her being in need of the most support, she still will look out for others more than herself. She used to host and cook for all friends and family, on regular occasions, which was a testament to how thoughtful and generous she is. She's still the same sister I grew up with and the jokes, banter and enjoyment of obnoxious metal music together hasn't changed.

So... back to me, Bex... I am not sure what the future holds for me. What will be will be.

10 Piece Unique

Nelleke Koeners and Axelle Herwyn

Nelleke, Mama Tars

On July 26, 1992, I became a mother for the first time, to a son. He was named Tars, after a Roman warrior from the 3rd century. Tars was a bit of a headstrong child. He observed everyone, and if he had a good feeling about you, you could be his friend. If not, he would completely ignore you.

Tars was very athletic, playing football for two teams and excelling in running. He was once tested at a high level to be coached as a long-distance runner, but Tars didn't like the discipline required for it—he wanted to become a chef instead. Nature also gave him a lot of energy; hunting and fishing were his passions, and he was a big animal lover. Our dog, chickens, geese, goats, and horses on our farm were his best friends and received all his attention and love.

Tars was also vain. His clothes had to be, as they say today, "Instagram-worthy." Despite this, he wasn't a very social boy and even earned the scout totem name "Lemon." When Tars was 12, he left for culinary school, over 100 kilometers away from our home. Tars lived in a boarding school to pursue his dream. He graduated successfully.

The Inseparable Duo (Written by Axelle, Tars' Girlfriend)

Tars and I met at a hotel school in Antwerp. We were both 16 years old at the time. We clicked immediately upon meeting. Tars' confidence and sense of humor instantly attracted me. A close friendship developed, full of fun and laughter, but also space for more serious conversations. Tars shared his dream of opening a restaurant one day, and he even had a name in mind: 'Piece Unique.' This summed him up perfectly because you wouldn't easily find someone more unique than Tars.

Before we knew it, we couldn't live without each other, and our friendship evolved into love. Two wonderful years went by, full of beautiful memories and unforgettable moments. Tars was someone with big dreams and even

DOI: 10.4324/9781003464181-10

bigger ambitions. After high school, he decided to study world cuisine in a specialization year at the best hotel school in Belgium. Together with three friends, they rented a nice apartment. Everything was falling into place, and he was so excited for what lay ahead… Just one more year of studying, and all his dreams could come true.

Mama Tars

It's now mid-September, and the 2010 school year started on Monday, September 19. On Sunday, September 26, 2010, we had dinner at my brother's house. Tars cooked, and around 7 p.m., he left to take his girlfriend home. Axelle said, "We held each other a bit longer than usual before he left, not knowing what would happen a few hours later."

Afterward, Tars drove to Koksijde, where the hotel school is, about 160 kilometers from our home. When he arrived, he and some friends went out for a drink. After a while, the boys, there were six of them, decided to go to one of their homes. They split into two cars, with Tars sitting behind the driver, wearing his seatbelt. None of the boys had been drinking. After about 700 meters of driving, they lost control of the car and crashed into a metal pole. The engine was found a distance away, and the speedometer was stuck at 90 km/h (on a road where the speed limit was 70 km/h). A passing car with a medical student stopped, and she immediately started CPR. At 2 a.m., the police came to our door with the terrible news about the accident. We left for the hospital right away, a 160-kilometer drive. In complete silence, I don't think Tars' father and I exchanged a word during the journey. Thousands of questions ran through our heads. We didn't know what had happened, only that Tars was severely injured.

September 26, 2010—A Day That Turned Our World Upside Down (Axelle)

It's Monday morning around half-past seven, and suddenly the phone rings. It's Tars' parents, telling me Tars has been in a very serious car accident and is critically injured. "He's currently undergoing surgery on his head… and he can't breathe on his own, he's on a ventilator. Prepare for the worst because things aren't looking good." Those words slowly started sinking in after a few minutes. I hung up and quickly told my parents and sister what was happening. Panic, sadness, a racing heart, and uncertainty took over. As an 18-year-old, I had no idea what awaited me. A few hours later, Tars' parents picked me up, and we drove to the hospital in Veurne. I had an hour and a half to think and gather my courage because I had no idea what would unfold.

Mama Tars

The ER doctor told us that Tars' brainstem was damaged and that as long as the bleeding continued, more vital functions would fail. They had placed Tars in a subcoma. After three days, the bleeding stopped, and after ten days, he started breathing on his own again.

Hospitals (Axelle)

The first encounter with the hospital is unforgettable. I can immediately visualize the sounds of the machines, the medication syringes next to Tars, and the room itself—I can even smell it. It's an image burned into my memory forever. After a while, the doctors called Tars' parents away to discuss his medical condition. I found myself standing alone next to my great love, who was going through so much, yet unaware of it. I didn't know what to say... I tried to reassure him by gently talking to him and touching him, so he knew he wasn't alone. Every day we stood by his side, shedding tears but also telling funny stories and sharing happy moments to make us laugh. I noticed that Tars' heart rate would increase when we entered the room and that his nostrils would flare. It was a rollercoaster. Some days were good for Tars, but others could take a turn for the worse.

Mama Tars

Tars remained in a coma and was transferred to a nursing home after about six weeks, where he was surrounded by elderly people. As his family (father, mother, brother, and girlfriend), we felt that Tars was trying to communicate with us, to reach out. But when we shared this with the doctors, they didn't believe us, telling us that we simply wanted to see something so badly that we were imagining it.

Axelle

Seeing that Tars was trying to connect with us gave us a glimmer of hope and renewed our determination to keep fighting. Days turned into weeks, and weeks turned into months. Tars was still in a coma, but I never doubted him or thought about giving up. I commuted daily between Veurne and home with the help of my parents, in-laws, and family, so I could spend 30 minutes with Tars in the evening. During the day, I went to school and worked hard to avoid needing extra time for assignments. Eventually, Tars was transferred to the Middelheim Hospital, where we could better monitor him—almost literally from our backyard. The doctors kept a close eye on Tars and informed us about steps being taken to make him as comfortable as possible.

Hospitals, after so many months, had no secrets for us, and sadly, it became a habit to spend hours there, sometimes from morning until night. Tars suffered from spasticity and fevers. It's a haunting memory to see him lying there covered in ice packs and heavily medicated to ease the pain. I wouldn't wish that uncertainty on anyone.

The character and willpower Tars had developed during all those months were invaluable. His strength held the family together, and none of us ever gave up. Giving up isn't in our vocabulary. Pushing through is.

Mama Tars

One day, while sitting at the dentist's office, I read an article in a magazine about Professor Steven Laureys and his Coma Science Group. I immediately contacted him, and in May 2012, we took Tars for a seven-day evaluation. The team had all kinds of medical equipment to measure brain activity, so after all the tests, they could determine the state of Tars' consciousness and how much brain activity was still present. Professor Laureys confirmed that Tars was a LIS (Locked-in Syndrome) patient. It was an unfamiliar term for us. Learning what LIS or Locked-in Syndrome meant was a relief, as it confirmed that our intuition had been right. From that moment on, we did everything we could to find a way to communicate with Tars. We started by having him blink to answer yes/no questions.

Neurologist, Doctor Steven Laureys (Axelle)

After some time, we came into contact with neurologist Dr. Steven Laureys. Tars was able to have a consultation in Liège, and several tests were scheduled. After these intense days, Tars was diagnosed with Locked-in Syndrome. He was fully conscious but unable to speak. In the first few years, there was little response when we spoke to him, or his reactions were extremely delayed. We were instructed to stimulate him as much as possible by continuing to communicate with him. After a while, I told him a joke, and I saw a small smile appear on his face. I can still remember that moment very well because I was so happy with something so small, yet at the same time, so big.

I refused to give up, which is why I gave my best every day. I talked to Tars, read to him, played his favorite music, and kept him updated on the things that had happened. I also found it important that he be involved in everything. In a way, we got to know and trust each other again. Tars knew very well that he should never feel ashamed or uncomfortable if something didn't work out right away. He had to feel safe in our little cocoon. Together, we found a new way to communicate through eye movements, and often, I only needed a glance to fully understand him. Not every day was easy, but his perseverance was admirable. Our bond grew even closer, and our love grew stronger, even in the silence. We enjoyed each other's company and learned that love doesn't always need words. Sometimes, it's in the small gestures toward one another.

Mama Tars

After Professor Steven Laureys' diagnosis, Tars had to return to the nursing home. For a 20-year-old to sit all day among the elderly, knowing that Tars understood everything, was difficult for us to accept as parents. We wanted to teach Tars more and help him further with rehabilitation so that he would at least be able to express himself. This was far from easy. Two years after the accident, there wasn't a single rehabilitation center that wanted to give Tars a chance. They all told us the same thing—that the first steps were always made in the first year and that things would stabilize after that, with only a very small chance of further development. It was maddening.

I personally had the best feeling about the K7 rehabilitation centre at the University Hospital, Ghent. I sent about 100 emails to the responsible doctor, called every week. I felt like a real stalker as a mother, but it worked. Dr. Annick Viaene said, "Why don't you come by with Tars?" And we did, successfully. She heard our cry for help and was willing to take Tars to the next level. Tars rehabilitated at K7 for 17 months, facing many obstacles—surgeries on his spastic feet, deformed wrists, and locked knees. In the first seven years after the accident, Tars was hospitalized 27 times, always with high fevers, lung and abdominal infections, or issues that puzzled the doctors. Five times, we received calls saying, "Come now, we think the end is near, Tars is dying."

Meanwhile, we searched for another solution to get Tars out of the nursing home. So Tars could come home on weekends, we had bought a car to transport him and even remodeled our house. Home is still, in our view, the best environment, and a familiar setting can work wonders. Fortunately, a new facility was built for young people with acquired brain injuries due to illness or accidents. There were only 20 rooms, but luck was on our side—Tars was welcome there. The building is near the water and the forest, an environment where Tars feels at home.

In 2017, a new rehabilitation center opened in Antwerp that works with different types of robotics. Another godsend. Since then, Tars has been going there twice a week to stay in shape. Thanks to this, he can now drive an electric wheelchair for about 20 minutes and hasn't been hospitalized since. Now, we're working on teaching him to communicate with a computer. It's not easy because Tars has limited concentration, but we keep trying. We're also teaching him to eat and drink again—everything works, but it's in small bites. It's been 14 years now, and we're still trying everything to give Tars the happiest life possible. Tars says he still finds life worth living.

14 Years Later (Axelle)

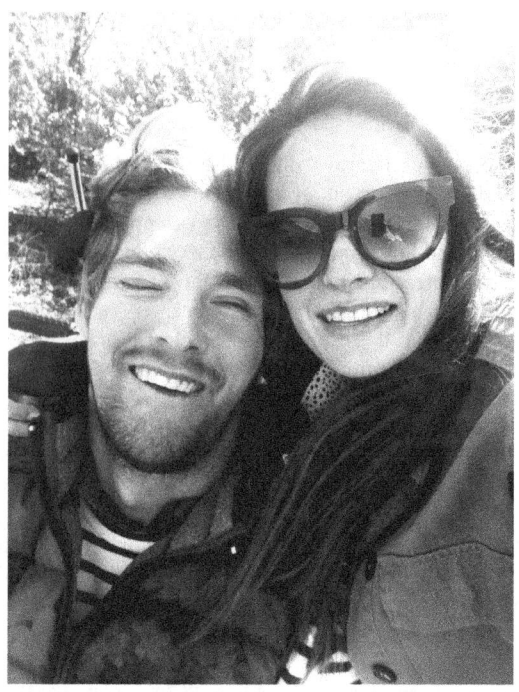

Tars and I have been together for 16 years now. We had envisioned our future very differently—there's no denying that. However, we've also had to travel a long road with many obstacles. Often, even today, I have to fight against prejudices. I've received too much "good" advice and comments that were completely out of place. Outsiders are often quick to impose their opinions and say things that can be extremely hurtful. They often assume they're right but don't consider someone else's feelings or thoughts. As a result, we've now surrounded ourselves only with people who truly care and with whom we feel safe, and above all, with whom we can be our true selves. Our circle of friends consists of a wonderful mix of women and men who are always there for us. We are never forgotten on important days, and they unconsciously always take us into account as a duo. The warmth we receive from them is indescribable.

Some time ago, one of Tars' best friends asked him if he wanted to be the godfather of their child. It was a beautiful moment to cherish. Tars and I spend weekends in our apartment, and those are such wonderful days that we both enjoy immensely. It may sound silly, but just like other people our age, we get to live together and simply be a couple. For others, that's a given, but not for us. Imagine not seeing or hearing your partner for days. We experience that, unfortunately, on a daily basis. That's why, after work, I often still drive to see Tars and enjoy time with just the two of us. I sometimes hear the comment, "Don't forget yourself, take some time for yourself," but then I ask, when was the last time you saw or heard your partner? And then the message sinks in. Everyone chooses how they view and navigate life.

Heartwarming (Axelle)

I want to thank my in-laws so much for involving me in this very special situation from day one. It means a lot to me that they understand the love between Tars and me. Even though we were still young at the time, they saw that we needed each other to keep growing and to get to where we are now. My in-laws and I had to get to know each other better in a short time, which was not easy, but I think the four of us have grown in a positive way.

I also want to mention my parents and family, who have supported me every second of every day in all the decisions I've made over the past few years and have been there for me whenever I needed them. I realize that's not a given. They may have had a different future in mind for their daughter, and I'm fully aware of that.

Perseverance (Axelle)

To those who find themselves in this "new" world, I want to give you some encouragement. You'll go through a very tough time, but remember, you're not alone. Nothing will be easy, as every situation is incredibly different and unique. But don't give up, and try to explore all possible paths. Get informed and don't be afraid to ask questions, so no one can take advantage of you. Stay positive and don't give up too quickly. You're stronger than you think. Keep the faith!

Mama Tars

On September 26, 2010, our lives were turned upside down in the blink of an eye. The world kept turning, but ours stood still. With ups and downs, with beautiful and less beautiful days, days of hope and despair. Days filled with laughter, but also days when tears were shed. Personally, I'm grateful that Tars has given me a new perspective—I now see the world in a different way. I'm deeply thankful that Tars has shown me, for more than 5,000 days, that each day is worth living.

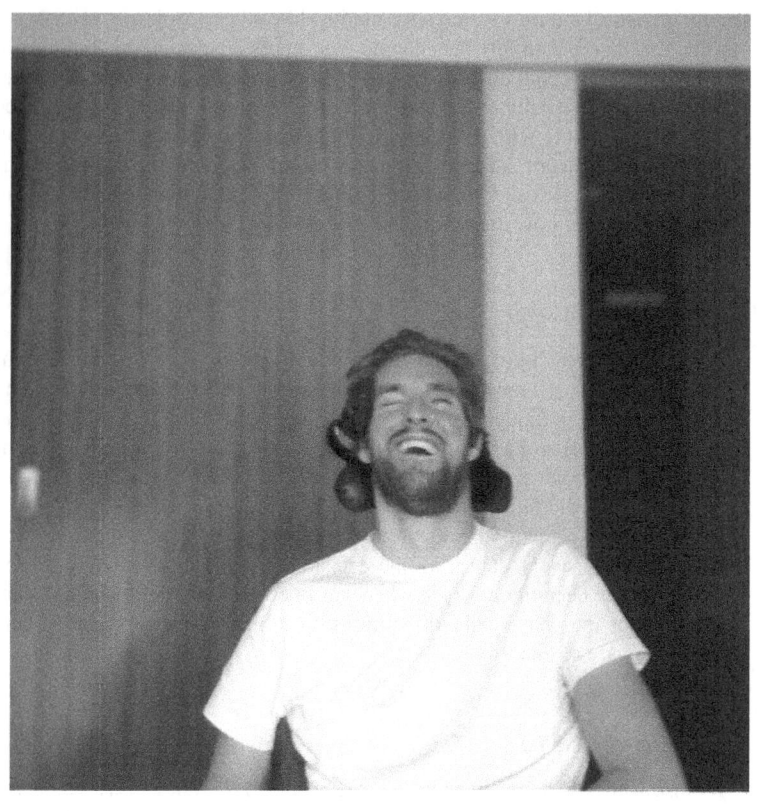

11 Let's Not Make a Whole Cheese Out of It

Isabelle Lauberthe

On October 31, 2008, I woke up feeling very tired, but it was hardly surprising; I had partied a little too hard the night before.

One of my friends had passed her nursing exam, and we had been celebrating all night long in the streets of Paris. As a Parisian, my life was completely in tune with the effervescence of the city.

Coming from a family with loving, caring parents and a very boisterous older brother, I grew up happy and carefree. After earning a degree in medicine and social work, I decided to study psychology at university, where I wanted to become a child psychiatrist. As things turned out, I became administrative director of an ophthalmology practice in the center of Paris.

I led an extremely active life, with a fascinating job, a happy and fulfilling relationship, and lots of outings with my friends.

And then came that fateful day of October 31, 2008.

I had taken the day off.

My partner and I had all sorts of commitments planned.

It was a very full day, somewhat clouded by an intense fatigue and an unusual, lasting weariness.

In the evening, the tiredness became associated with a very severe headache and tingling in my entire left arm. My partner called the emergency medical service. I spoke to the doctor who told me to go to the hospital. Overwhelmed by the exhaustion, the headache, and the tingling, I decided to go back to bed, saying "We'll see tomorrow!", convinced that nothing could happen to me, at 35 years old and in perfect health.

It was a terrible night.

Early in the morning, I sat down on the bed to go to the toilet and rolled over onto my left side. I couldn't sit up again. My partner suddenly realized the seriousness of the situation.

He sent for a doctor, who immediately had me hospitalized.

It was November 1st, a public holiday in France. I spent the entire day in an examination room, watching a parade of doctors who repeatedly performed the same tests on me, over and over again. From time to time, my partner managed to come and see me and say a few reassuring words. At around 7 pm,

DOI: 10.4324/9781003464181-11

I was asked if I agreed to undergo an MRI. We were trying to have a child, so it would be dangerous if I were pregnant. I immediately agreed. I caught a glimpse of my mother, who would tell me years later that I kept asking the time, and that my mouth was twisted. After the MRI, I underwent a series of lumbar punctures and other tests.

It was late, we were in a corridor waiting to be transferred to another hospital. I was lying on a stretcher, stroking my partner's hair. All of a sudden, he burst into tears, burying his face in my stomach. It was at that moment that I realized what was happening was serious. I was taken to another hospital. I saw a whole bunch of caregivers rushing towards me. They used incomprehensible terms and handled me from all sides.

Suddenly, I felt an intense pain in my throat. This would be my last memory of November 1st, 2008.

I woke up not knowing exactly how much time had passed. According to my parents, it had been a day. I felt as if I were in a semi-reality. I oscillated between moments of lucidity and hallucinations. Sometimes I thought I was in a hospital in the United States, or in a laboratory in Germany.

I saw people around me, I tried to call out to them but no sound came out of my mouth. I saw I had tubes everywhere, but one was particularly unpleasant and irritating. It was the one at the back of my throat, the one that allowed me to breathe.

My partner and my parents were omnipresent. I had so many unanswered questions. I saw people bustling all around me. Some talked to me, others didn't even see me. I had no bearings. I didn't know where I was, what was happening to me, I had the feeling I was losing myself. I spent countless

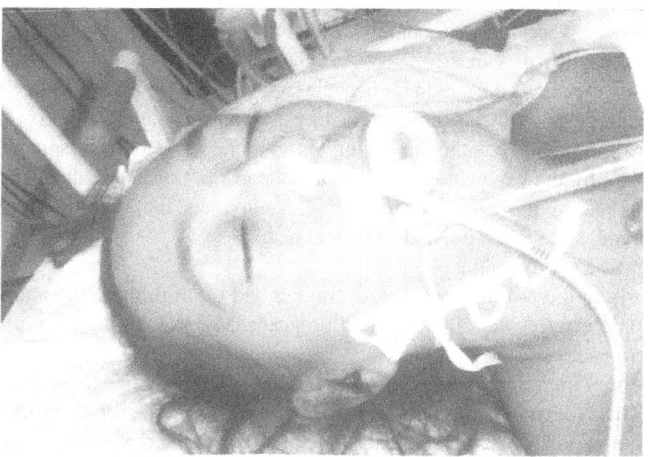

Figure 11.1 November 2, 2008.

hours, probably days, going over the same questions. But when I addressed people, they never answered me. I could see that I could no longer speak, no longer move, but it immediately plunged me into a deep torpor and my analytical mind was completely disoriented. The daily visits of my partner and parents were my only comfort and reference point.

One day, a very kind doctor approached me and explained that a board with the letters of the alphabet would be put in place so that I could communicate with the outside world. My partner had noticed that I was trying to express myself through my gaze and had mentioned it to the care team. When the doctor suggested this board, an incredible feeling of happiness washed over me from head to toe. The alphabet was arranged according to the most frequently used letters. With a blink of an eye, I would validate the desired line, then at the announcement of the desired letter, I would blink again. It would be long and tedious, but this board would become my salvation. Often, throughout the day, blinking became difficult and my concentration was hard to maintain! This earned me a number of arguments with my partner.

One night, I was lying askew and my back was hurting terribly. Having no way to alert the caregivers, I realized that if I cried, it would cause a pulmonary congestion and the saturometer alarm would go off, forcing a nurse to come in. So I started crying (for many reasons), the alarm went off as expected and a nurse entered. I signaled to her with my eyes to take my board so that I could spell out 'BACK'. She looked at my board and said, 'Oh! Your thing, I don't understand it!' She left, turning off the light and closing the door. At that moment, my physical pain was coupled with an indescribable psychological suffering. That night was one of the worst of my life.

Gradually, they tried to sit me up in a large, comfortable wheelchair, strapped in with sheets to prevent me from falling forward. The first few times weren't very successful, as after a few minutes I had to be laid back down due to severe dizziness. I was able to stop using the ventilator and instead had a tracheostomy. I also had a nasal feeding tube for nutrition, hydration, and medication, but this was later replaced with a tube directly into my stomach. At that time, it was unimaginable to consider continuing my life. Unfortunately, I had no way of stopping this new life that was being imposed on me. I did try asking my partner for help, but he flatly refused. In hindsight, I agree with his decision!

One day, my parents were allowed to take me for a walk around the hospital grounds in my big, comfy VIP chair. They wanted to take me to the cafeteria downstairs. The elevator arrived and they pushed my wheelchair inside. Facing the mirror, I saw a bloated woman, with a hole in her throat, disheveled hair, and a lifeless body. I screamed—internally. The shock was so overwhelming that I couldn't even spell the word 'MIRROR' on my board. My parents and the people around me wondered why I was in such a desperate state. It took me several minutes to explain to my parents. I hadn't seen myself in months, and the shock was terrible!

Following this incident, the speech therapist had me work in front of a mirror every day. Speech therapy was particularly difficult as I couldn't do any of the exercises. Opening my mouth, sticking out my tongue—nothing was possible. I enjoyed physical therapy more, although it was only passive mobilization.

One evening, I asked my partner to give me a pen to write with because I was tired of spelling everything out. He said no, it wasn't possible. I repeated my request, emphasizing it with irritated blinks, but he refused again. He then got up and left the room without a word, leaving me annoyed and puzzled. Two minutes later, I saw him return accompanied by a doctor. At that moment, I cursed him, thinking he had gone to complain about me. The woman came up to me and asked if I wanted a pen to write with. I closed my eyes in agreement, and she replied very gently, 'But miss, it's not possible, you can't move anymore!' At those words, my eyes fell on my hands, which remained completely still despite all my efforts to move them. The inner pain I felt was indescribable. It was as if a bomb had exploded inside me. Even 15 years later, I can still feel fragments of that harsh reality. I don't know why I still hadn't realized that I was completely paralyzed. Perhaps it was a bit of denial that made me believe some possibilities still existed. My boss would regularly visit me, but on that day, for the first time, I refused to see him. I was too devastated.

I spent 6 months in intensive care. 6 months constantly hooked up to machines. 6 months being fed and hydrated through a tube. It took them a long time to make a diagnosis. After weeks of tests, the results finally came in—a foodborne bacterium, listeriosis, had nestled itself 'invisibly' in my brainstem and then began its ascent. It was after six weeks that it dealt the final blow. The night of October 31st was my official encounter with LISTERIA. The damage caused during the incubation period is dramatic and irreversible. This bacterium can be found in uncooked foods or raw milk cheese. For there to be consequences, a large quantity of the food must be ingested. I therefore had to recall the so-called sensitive foods I had eaten six months prior. After many hours of reflection and mental anguish, I remembered a cheese I had eaten in large quantities during my vacation in the South of France. I will never know for sure if this cheese was 100% responsible for my collapse, but I have strong suspicions and a real gut feeling about it.

One day, I was told I would have to go to a hospital with a rehabilitation center. This was to be my new home for the next 18 months. On the second day, the nurses wheeled a stretcher into my room and told me 'go to the shower!' It had been 6 months since I had only had bed baths. Suddenly, I was terrified of the idea of having a jet of water on my body! Everything was a source of apprehension, but above all the fear of being drowned! Which, of course, was totally ridiculous. Eventually, I came to appreciate this moment on the shower stretcher and whenever it crossed the threshold of my room, I felt a great deal of joy.

In the ward, there was quite intensive rehabilitation with, every day: physiotherapy, orthopedics, occupational therapy, and psychomotor therapy. The only small problem was that my physiotherapist was visually impaired and I was almost mute. In terms of understanding, we sometimes ran into our own limits. However, I was able to work intensively and regain some movements like grasping with my right hand or standing upright with a support in front of me. A hyperextension of the knees (recurvatum) allows me to stand. My knees lock once I am standing. Walking would be impossible, but being able to stand upright is very useful as it has many benefits. Walking is no longer a priority. The essential thing is to be able to function in the most effective way possible. I met a fantastic occupational therapist who taught me to adapt using the aids available to me. She made me a unicorn to help me read. It's a plastic rod with a non-slip piece at the end that is to be attached around the forehead to turn the pages of a book, using the mobility of the head. It takes a lot of patience and determination to achieve this. Over the years, I regained some mobility in my right hand and I can now read "normally", although turning the pages is still tedious.

And then there was a speech therapist. I think it was the first beautiful and great encounter of my new life. This man, through his patience, professionalism, and humanism, taught me every day to eat again and to express myself. A spoonful of compote or puree could take 40 minutes to swallow. With his patience and my determination, we repeated this learning process on a daily basis for months. Little by little it became two spoons, then three. When I talk about it today, I wonder how I managed to keep going through this ordeal over and over again. I think I became a "performer"—my life was the ring and I was becoming a fighter. Every small progress became a great victory. Every noon, I could smell the meal trays, which was extremely painful but at the same time it was a motivation to succeed. For a very long time, I continued with my daily spoonfuls. After about a year, my tracheotomy was removed. The removal of this cannula in my throat was a real joy and pride! I could start eating "per os" (by mouth) again, but my diet was exclusively pureed. It was only after 5 years that my diet became "almost normal", but to this day I still avoid certain foods considered "difficult" (rib-eye steaks for instance). I was also able to drink again but in the form of gelled water for many years.

I eventually returned to liquids, sparkling water exclusively, although I am still prone to a few persistent but controlled mishaps.

As far as speaking was concerned, I could express myself through sounds and then words, by associating them with movements of my eyelids to agree or disagree. Little by little, the wonderful occupational therapist found ways to try to make me move my right arm. All sensitivity in my left side had disappeared. For the record, I was left-handed! As a result, I had to relearn everything on my right side. From wheelchair to wheelchair, I learned to drive an electric one, which was a giant leap towards independence. It was a real freedom that I quickly got used to.

I stayed there for a year and a half. I knew everyone, people appreciated me for who I had become. My room had become my den. The walls were covered with photos, maps, and drawings. I had an extra clothes rack added. Every noon, my parents would come and bring me coffee that we would thicken with powder. My partner also came every day. Over the months, the visits became more diverse: colleagues, friends, family. Each first time was a profound upheaval. From time to time, I was allowed to go out on Sundays. It was on a transport voucher intended for the paramedics that I first saw the words 'Locked-In Syndrome'. Having read Mr. Bauby's book "The Diving Bell and the Butterfly", I immediately knew what they referred to. Months went by as I went through weekly rehabilitation sessions, regular visits, and Sunday outings. The apartment where we lived was not wheelchair accessible, so my outings took place at my parents' house. My partner found a suitable flat a short time later. Going back to the hospital on Sunday evenings was difficult, for I did not want to leave my partner. Yet ultimately, this life protected by the hospital walls and the kindness of the caregivers suited me perfectly. But one day, a big meeting took place with all the therapists and my family and partner to announce that I had to go home. A feeling of apprehension coupled with a fear of the unknown immediately came over me. I was going to have to face this new life stuck in a wheelchair and 100% dependent. During this meeting, they mentioned the need to have home care assistants. I knew nothing about their role and their immeasurable presence.

The occupational therapist came to our new home to recommend some adaptations. She suggested we replace our bed with a medical one. I firmly refused, as it would have a negative impact on the relationship with my partner. However, after the first night in our apartment, I requested a double medical bed because I couldn't physically sleep on our old one anymore. My days revolved around physical therapy, speech therapy, and care from home health aides. The words I could pronounce turned into sentences, and I was able to make more and more facial expressions to my speech therapist. Life as a couple had changed drastically. My partner juggled the shortcomings of the home care agency, my difficulty accepting my new situation, and the challenges inherent in disability. As the years went by, our life together became increasingly unmanageable. I think for a long time, he believed he could save me with his love, but unfortunately his efforts were in vain. Everything became unbearable for him. In 2012, he decided to leave. His decision was very difficult to accept, but I will never allow myself to judge him for it. For me, living with illness is an obligation. For him, it was a choice. Unable to support myself financially, I moved to Paris and ended up settling near my parents. My partner's departure forced me to become more independent in terms of organization and administration. I had to take charge of my new life. My days, months, and years evolved through my encounters. I rediscovered ordinary

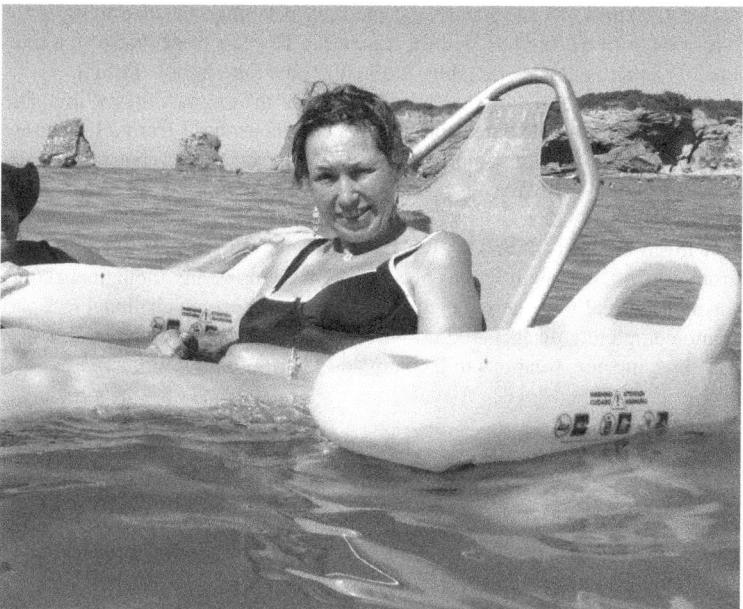

Figure 11.2 My first time on the Tiralo.

things that became extraordinary. One of the most striking examples is my first swim in the sea, 6 years after my body stopped functioning. It was during my first vacation at a rehabilitation center. There is a special kind of floating loungers called a Tiralo.

The first time I was laid on them, I felt an incredible mix of fear, joy, stress, and happiness coming over me. It was a real tsunami that overturned my heart. And then there were the trips, to the Dominican Republic, Mexico (for my 10th anniversary as a wheelchair user) and Marrakech. Over the years, I've made wonderful encounters and savored every moment of happiness to the fullest.

It takes time to realize the incredible luck of having two lives in one…

It's been 15 years and I know with absolute clarity that the fight will never be over.

Accepting my total dependence and the necessary help of carers.

Forgiving the harshness of certain words or looks that make people so hateful but which, in most cases, stem from ignorance and misunderstanding.

Overcoming difficulties and obstacles for a minimum of pleasure.

So I decided to embrace motivation and willpower, making them as much a part of me as my disability.

I don't know if I have truly accepted my disability, but one thing is for sure, I have learned to live with it. It took me 11 years to get back on a tram and 14 years to get back on a bus. No matter how long it took, I did it.

I feed on projects and challenges. They are the engines of my life. The obstacles are numerous, the shortcomings enormous, but I learn a little more each day that I shouldn't look back and ask myself "why," but rather look forward and say "why not."

My heart has gained what I have lost in mobility.

I loved my first life madly, but I much prefer the person I have become. From now on, my small battles become great victories, my thoughts become ways of living, I meet heroic people and my goals become challenges. A part of me completely disappeared on November 1st, 2008, but this annihilation has given me new weapons to face my new, extra-ordinary life.

12 A Brainstem Stroke which Led to Locked-in Syndrome

Wenche Loseth

My name is Wenche, and I am from Ulsteinvik in Norway. I had a brainstem infarction that resulted in Locked-in Syndrome, and I ended up in this situation on March 8, 2000. I need help with most practical things in my daily life. It has been a journey to get to the everyday life I have today!

No one around me in the acute phase expected anything from me, especially the hospital staff. My family had hope. One day, my mother sat and looked at me. She looked me in the eyes and said, "Squeeze your eyes shut if you can hear me?" I squeezed my eyes shut with all my strength! That was when my family rejoiced, and contact was established. It took two years before I moved home. My husband had prepared most things for me.

I live my life with my family, my three daughters, and their children, and I live in my own house, gradually reclaiming the roles I lost on that March day in 2000. I got divorced three months after I moved home. It hasn't been easy with the municipality regarding the primary help I should receive.

I have focused on the future because I can influence it – the past is already lived and can't be changed.

To take control of my everyday life, the word "threshold" came up the very first week I moved back home. This applied to both people coming in and out. My home and my body have become others' workplaces. Everyone wanted to help me and meant well. The support system that was supposed to be established around me, especially the home care service, planned the help they would give me based on their own needs! They didn't think of me, and certainly not my family. My youngest daughter was 9 years old.

I didn't dare protest at first, out of politeness. I accepted most things because I didn't dare to do otherwise.

To the municipality, I was a "patient" who was incapable of making my own decisions. They hadn't even familiarized themselves with my needs! I didn't know much about my situation either. I couldn't find anything online. The only thing I was sure of was that I knew what I wanted. Maybe that was enough?

This was my starting point.

I quickly realized I had to start somewhere. I had a switch installed that I could handle for my front door, so I could open it myself, preferably when it

DOI: 10.4324/9781003464181-12

suited me! Then I forced myself out. First to meet the villagers, then everyone else. I had been home on leave quite often, so I knew a little about the paths here.

Then I began working with the municipality to make them understand that I wanted and intended to live. I actually wanted to reclaim the life roles I had before! Especially having responsibilities as a parent. My family and children were not a topic for the support system. The words about all this were there. Holistic! But the practice was something completely different.

The municipality wanted to give me care to survive in a way that suited them, which I didn't want. I wanted help to live. This was many years ago, but I know many still struggle with such attitudes in the support system today and will continue to "fight" with this "system" for many years to come.

I have gradually received BPA (citizen-controlled personal assistance) during the day and evening. In the evenings and at night, I use home care services. I find it good to have contact with healthcare personnel because I need it occasionally. I have chosen this solution myself because it allows me to have some time to myself during the day. I have been clear about how I wanted things all along. I have found that if I am clear, it is easier for the support system to work towards the same goals with me.

This is what is normal for me now. I have many foreign hands all over my skin, but I let no one under my skin. That's where my private life is, to the extent I have one.

I have worked hard not to become bitter. It took many years before I could see myself as a resource and not a burden to others. The adjustment processes are ongoing, and I am reminded every day of what I have lost. I can't get used to what happened to me, that's just how it is.

I use the "Donald Duck method" when dealing with mental issues; when negative thoughts come, I run them over with positive thoughts. I use the scales and let the heavier side be positive and keep the focus there. It's not easy when the choices in everyday life are often between the plague and cholera.

The setbacks come from time to time, usually caused by things I can't influence. I can usually get back up again, but the margins are small, and things can easily create a domino effect.

When the public sector introduces new rules, restructuring, and reforms, I am usually the one who has to adapt to the regulations and institutions I depend on, in addition to finding new solutions in my everyday life. This often applies from the highest level of medical expertise to the most basic services in the municipality. I am often the one left alone with the challenges.

I experienced becoming "a case in the system" when this happened. At first, I didn't reflect on it. I started to miss my name, my identity! The system segregated me from the concept of being human! Among other things, by calling me a "patient" at all times. They always want someone with me when anyone is to talk to me, no matter if it concerns my private life.

I also began reacting to how many people were speculating and expressing opinions about me, often about things I found very private.

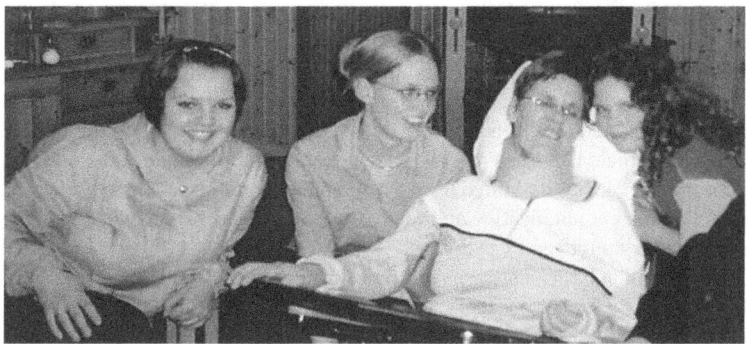

Figure 12.1 This is me and my daughters. Arleen on the left, Siw Elise in the middle, and Ann Kristin on my right. This photo was taken at Ålesund Hospital during the acute phase.

Three to four months after I moved home again, I received a meeting report from the municipality. The home care personnel had had a staff meeting – essentially about my private life. I felt ill. The letter made me realize how exposed I had become. Even my preference for certain clothes was referenced because they were focused on what was easiest for them.

I constantly use a lot of resources to protect myself. To safeguard both my and my family's integrity.

I have seen changes over the years. Among other things, my municipality is more flexible and better accommodates my needs today. My experience is that the NAV reform is much better than the old system. The digital development has made my life much easier and contributed to a much more private life. Not least, the development of aids. That has been extremely difficult.

When I am out, I meet many people who don't quite trust me and are unsure. My voice doesn't inspire confidence in people. Everyone sees my disability! But what's between my ears, people don't see – it can be both embarrassing and amusing when people try to figure it out! The people I meet in my daily life are "ordinary people." "Ordinary people" are not specialists in communication and disabilities. I don't think anyone can expect that.

Rehabilitation institutions need to think more about this. Prepare people who are going "out" to live their lives again in society.

My fellow citizens perceive me very differently since this happened to me. It's not meant to be harmful; most are sympathetic on my behalf. "Ordinary people" don't understand that I am the same as I was before.

A clear example of this is driving. No one can understand that I drive with my driver's license, which I got when I was 18! Everyone assumes I took a new license after the stroke! Many associate a stroke with forgetting one's past and life experience. I am not the exception, especially when people hear my voice, even though they understand everything I say! Sometimes I don't use my voice. Simply to avoid having to prove that I am trustworthy.

I don't handle my voice very well. In my head, I still have my old voice, my quick wit and speed, but I hear the sounds coming out of my mouth. I do use my voice. But I can't bear to listen to it myself through, for example, recordings. I get sick and often have a drop in blood pressure. The importance of facilitating communication and following up on the loss of my voice seems to have gone unnoticed by everyone.

My situation has changed several times over the years, both positively and negatively. The support systems struggle to adapt to my changes, even when I inform them. In the first few years, I felt like a burden to most who were supposed to help me. That I had become a burden to society as a whole. Many can bring out that feeling in me with the way they speak to me. The major NAV reform has made my daily life easier as it has settled in.

There were several reasons I chose to write a book about all I had experienced. Once I made that decision, I sat down to remove everything I had written that I didn't dare to share. Everything that could be recognized by someone was removed. The community here where I live is small. I still have to live and stay here.

Help and accommodation for communication have not been prioritized in my municipality or the assistive technology center I am affiliated with.

I have had to manage communication on my own all these years. Even though I've asked for help many times, it seems like it hasn't been taken seriously.

Losing my voice has been the most difficult part of my situation. I often feel "overridden" by others in this area. I communicate with my voice, eyes, and head movements. I usually use email to communicate with strangers. Unfortunately, I've experienced many instances of "communication violations." These violations are the worst part of my daily life. For example, someone might ask me 6-7 questions at once! I manage to take a breath, and then the person has moved on!

Some of these instances have been so severe that I've had to address them afterward. I've also learned and experienced how to "prevent" unpleasant situations. I had a baclofen pump implanted in 2003, which is crucial for controlling spasms and has been so over the years.

No one is allowed to touch my body before communication with the person who is going to help me has been established. This way, I can explain what I need help with and be prepared for the activity that follows. It's easy for staff to become "too familiar" with my body. But it's my body!

I have had many thoughts and asked myself many questions over the years! I believe that's just how it is.

I've loved exercising my whole life, which has helped me in this situation. After six years of intense training, I managed to walk independently with the help of a walker. This has made my daily life much easier. I stand up and walk several times a day. To date, I have approximately 22,000 hours of intense physical training outside of my wheelchair. It's the best spasm control I can get! My "biggest hurdle" is asking my helper: can you go get my walker? I feel much better in every way when I train every day. I haven't reached my goals, as they were probably too high, but I didn't know what to expect. I've trained hard to regain my voice and the ability to eat through my mouth again. I see training opportunities in everything I do. I've learned that limitations are often mental. A lack of motivation motivates me even more. I've noticed that it's motivating for my support system as well.

I walk using a walker that is customized for me, with an assistant walking behind to support me. Sometimes, I use a regular climbing harness. I've fallen many times but getting up from the floor is manageable. I've planned for the occasional fall. I have a good support system today, but ultimately, it's me who has to do the work.

The most important thing for me is to spend my everyday life with my family – that is my "everyday rehabilitation." Without my family, I wouldn't have managed so well or lived in my own house.

There wasn't any support system for us as a family when we needed it most. Holistic rehabilitation was not practiced in my municipality 24 years ago. Nor did I experience family being a focus at the rehabilitation institution. My family has followed me every step of the way, through both ups and downs. It has been difficult for my family. I think at times it's been tougher for my daughters than for me. There was no support system for children when this happened to me. My family was shocked by what happened to me. Everyone in the family mourns the "loss" of me, and they have to live with that too. Over time, I have reclaimed my everyday life and my roles. In my mind, it has been a given that I wouldn't just survive, but live. Today, I see that my daughters use the experience they have gained with me in their daily lives and education in a positive way. We've had several tough events in my family in recent years. But we have managed well and used the experience we've gained to cope with most things.

I write a lot about my experiences. I've written about all kinds of topics ranging from euthanasia to living without my voice. I find writing to be good therapy. I've learned how important this is. The family also needs to be taken care of, perhaps more than anything else. I've achieved my goal of creating the home and base my daughters need. It's the most important thing in my life. We've walked a path that has been very difficult and tough. It has made us very close in our daily lives. Two of my daughters live in the neighborhood. You can do what you want when you want to do what you can.

When it comes to the accessibility of services, especially those with confidentiality, I've been frustrated. The staff I've encountered in these situations have made things worse, particularly by shouting out sensitive information. Many people think I'm deaf as well. It's distressing to have to call before an event to ask if I can get in. Most of the time, I can't.

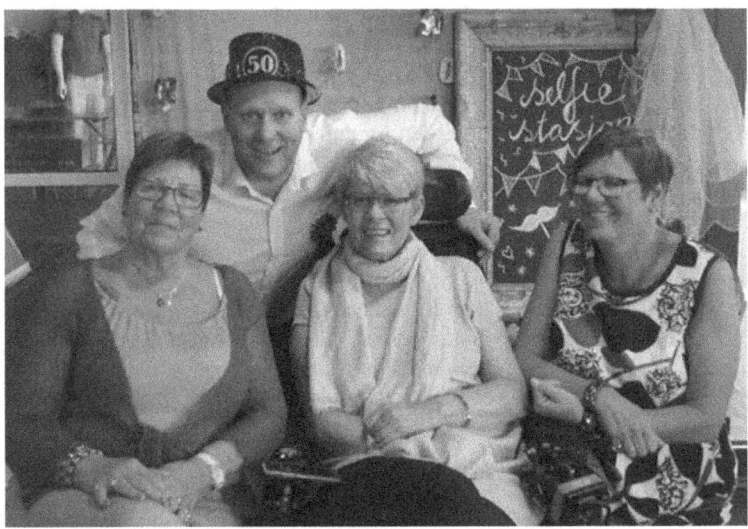

Figure 12.2 My mother Aud, my brother Geir Oskar, and my sister Hege.

My mother, brother, and sister have walked this journey with me. So did my late father. The entire family was affected when I suffered a brainstem stroke in 2000.

I'm a grandmother to William, Tale, Isabel, Nicholas, Edel, and Olivia. My grandchildren love the mountains, outdoor activities, and handball. They've never known anything other than that their grandmother is in a wheelchair. I was already paralyzed by the brainstem stroke when the grandchildren were born.

I'm proud of that because I've hiked many places across the country, played handball for 30 years, and skied a lot. We are a sports-loving family. My daughters, grandchildren and I are all involved in sports. We spend a lot of quality time in the sports hall. Handball is the favorite and we are three generations of goalkeepers for Hødd Handball.

What could I expect of myself? How long will I live? What is it like to grow old in such a situation? Can I compare myself to anyone? What should I prioritize? What is best for me? No one has been able to answer all my questions over these years!

I often ask myself where I find the motivation for everything in my daily life! Especially on days when the spasms twist my muscles in every direction while the arthritis and headaches take their toll. My experience is that most of it is mental, no matter what I try. The spasms that affect all my muscles are constantly changing and controlling most things. I've been fortunate to have the same people around me all these years who help me with the spasms. They know me well, and I receive good treatment. The setbacks have been tough,

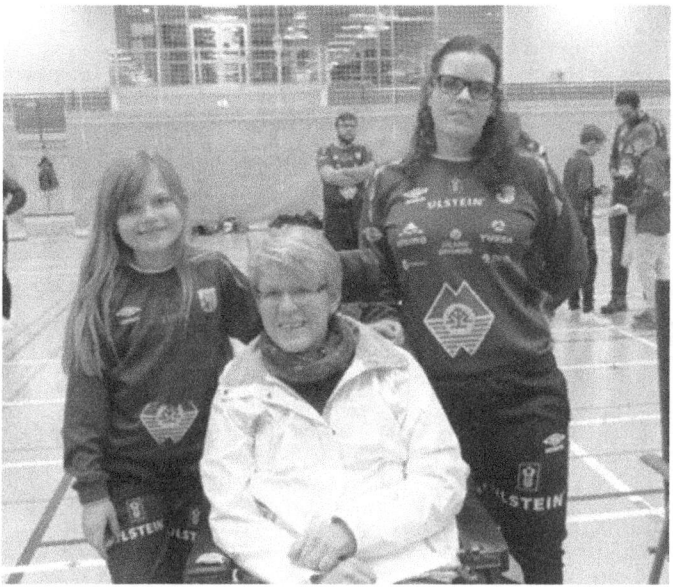

Figure 12.3 Isabel, my granddaughter, Ann Kristin, my daughter, and I together in the sports hall.

often caused by circumstances I can't influence or control myself. At times, it has taken up to a year to train myself back to where I was.

I drive my car with a joystick and have done so since 2005. The reason I wanted to do this is a long story. But I knew it was possible. Car issues are often complex and can take a long time. So I started the process immediately. They've made significant advancements in adapting the driving environment in cars. In August 2018, I received my new car. Over these 19 years, there has been progress that is hard to comprehend! I can't imagine a day without the ability to drive myself!

Regarding assistive devices in general, there has been incredible progress. But at the same time, constant changes in rules and regulations can make it very exhausting. The biggest challenge with assistive devices is the time you have to wait after the need arises! It's the same challenge when it comes to repairing assistive devices!

There is some planning involved before a trip, but good planning makes the trip more successful! I found out that traveling is fine by doing a trial run. I need to bring the best wheelchair I have. I've discovered that flights of about five hours are the longest I can handle without getting too tired. The trip can be long, but I have to calculate the hours without the wheelchair to determine if I can take the trip.

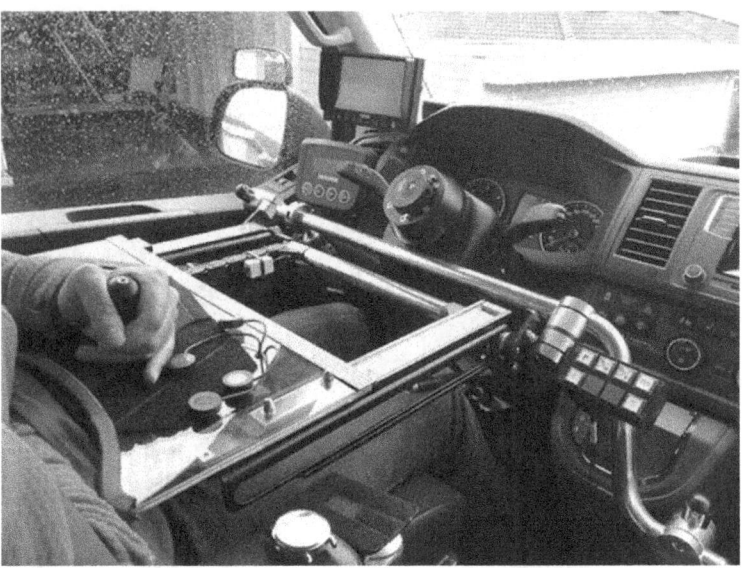

Figure 12.4 Me driving my car, here is my new car that I got in 2018.

I worked two days a week for nine years, including work training. I worked in a shared administration for several kindergartens – of course, using a computer as my tool. I stopped working in the fall of 2013.

I realized that working a little could be very beneficial. I had the support of some people who believed in me. It was Aetat (the employment service) at the time. They didn't get involved until the end, and there's a long story behind that.

I've given many lectures about various experiences in several places around the country – mostly on Sunnmøre.

Today, I partially live off the art I create. I paint pictures with my mouth, which I started doing in 2011 by chance. Someone thought it would be good training for my neck. I must admit I was a bit surprised myself on the first try.

I've held three exhibitions at home in Ulsteinvik.

In my "previous" professional life, I mainly worked at the largest shipyard in Ulstein. I've had my commitments, especially in sports, music, and outdoor activities. Not least as a parent! Life experiences that I haven't forgotten.

I create strategies to try and achieve the goals I set for myself. Sometimes I have to give up, but then I try a new strategy! When resignation comes, I can experience it positively. Because then I feel my shoulders relax, and I can use the resources it frees up for other things!

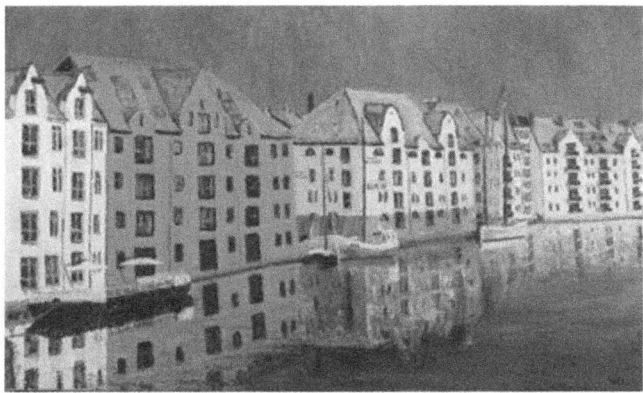

Figure 12.5 This painting is of Brosundet in Ålesund, and it's the largest I've ever painted. I painted it right after a trip to Spain. At that time, my body was relaxed and flexible, including my neck and jaw.

I have received some column space back home in Sunnmøre. On those occasions, I have been able to focus on many things, especially in terms of accessibility, inclusion, attitudes towards being affected by a stroke, and preconceived notions!

I have been able to focus on the "boxing in" of myself and others.

I have also spoken out in reader contributions and replies in the local newspaper. I rarely do that, but when I have, it has been warranted! I have experienced in those situations that it is worthwhile to speak up!

Maybe it's the first wheelchair on Breifjellet on Hareidlandet? A fantastic experience and a goal achieved! Unfortunately, I didn't make it all the way to the top. The last slope was too steep. Not for me, but for the terrain chair. It completely stopped and would only go backward. It was a strenuous but enjoyable trip.

In 2010, on my own initiative, I attended a conference in Germany on Locked-in Syndrome. For the first time, I received information and learned more about the brainstem stroke I had suffered from. I finally got to meet people who live with this condition. No professional agency has ever explained to me what kind of stroke I have had. Ellen Høyer, who is a neuro-physiotherapist at Sunnaas Hospital, handed the book I wrote to Dr. Karl-Heinz Pantke, who is from Germany and has done a lot of research on this type of stroke. He was one of the organizers of the conference I attended. This diagnosis affects one person per four million people per year.

One of the most important goals I have had is to live in my own home and be a mother. It has been a journey to reach the relatively free life I have today. I understand those who want to give up. But living my everyday life with my family, that I have managed. I AM the same person I always have been, but

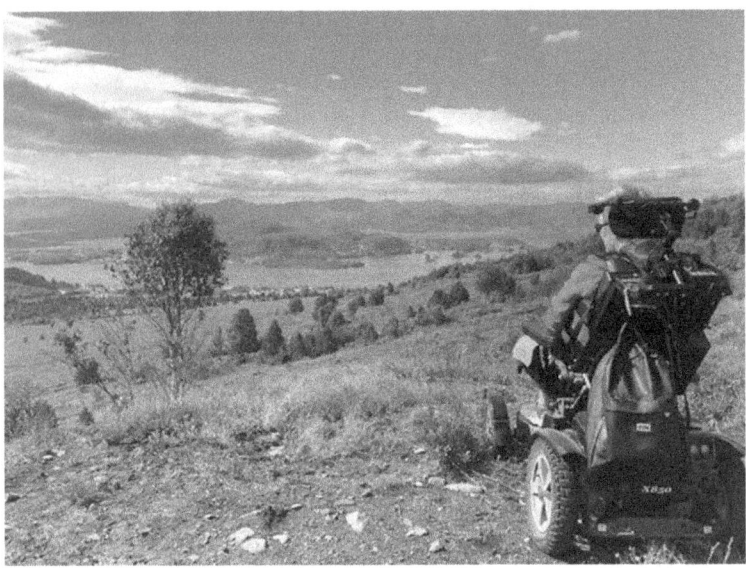

Figure 12.6 Me on the mountain in Sunnmøre.

I HAVE acquired a serious disability. My doors are open all day for my three daughters, and they come to me when they need me. That's how it should be. I am glad that I have been healthy, independent, and have had the opportunity to use my creativity. I decided early on that I want to be a resource for my family, not a burden. Being able to see myself in this way has been time-consuming. Most of it is, and has been, tough processes to get through. It's going well!

Seize the day. Seize the moment. My own legs have carried me to the top many times. Beautiful and a beauty for the soul, combined with sorrow and loss. That's life.

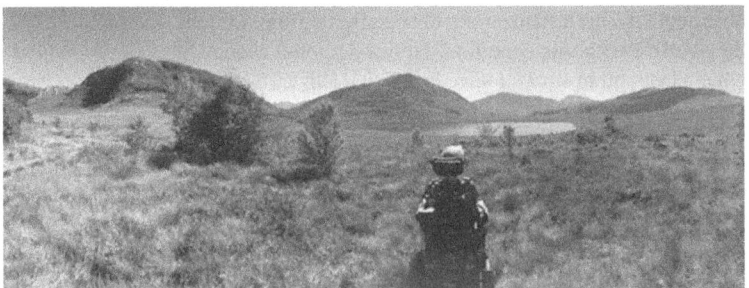

13 Light at the End of the Road

Paqui Villegas, translated by Fernando Vidal

My name is Paqui Villegas, I'm from La Mamola, a village in the province of Granada, Andalusia (Spain). I currently live in a residence for persons with severe disabilities in the capital city of Almería, close to my hometown. I am 54 years old, and I suffer from LIS (Locked-In Syndrome). In these lines, I will share my personal experience, with the intention of bringing some light for those who have suffered a stroke like me, or any traumatic setback in their lives, and who currently feel lost. My goal is to help them see a future perspective full of hope and excitement.

My story begins on October 17, 2008. At that time, I was 39 years old, and one could say my life was in order; I had a steady job, a home, a car, a stable relationship, and felt that I had a complete life, possessing everything any person my age could desire. I was completely happy.

I have always considered myself as an active and very optimistic person. I enjoyed sports and paid moderate attention to my eating habits. I loved always being surrounded by friends and family. I was a very cheerful and outgoing person, always looking at the bright side of things. I had never suffered from a serious illness, just an occasional headache. But one day, everything changed.

I remember feeling strange that week. Every day, I felt pain in my neck, but I thought it was because of work. After all, who hasn't had a sore neck once in a while? The pain persisted, so one afternoon, I went to the emergency doctor for a check-up. He only diagnosed me with a bit of torticollis [a painful condition that causes the neck to twist and the head to tilt], and prescribed something for the pain and told me to rest. After a while, I felt a terrible pain in my neck, and I noticed that I was starting to lose balance. I barely managed to call my closest family member. They didn't quite understand what I was saying because they noticed I had difficulty coordinating my words. Then I fell down, vomited, and lost consciousness. When I woke up in hospital, I was bewildered. I didn't understand why I was there, and I tried to get up, but my body wouldn't respond. I couldn't move a single muscle; I was completely paralyzed and unable to speak.

DOI: 10.4324/9781003464181-13

I felt heavily sedated. As I later found out, I was in the ICU for five days. I could barely open my eyes; I just wanted to sleep. I had a moment of clarity and thought, "What has happened to me? How long am I going to be like this? Why did this happen to me? Why do I have a tube in my mouth to breathe?" You sink, you cry, you think, "I can't stand seeing myself like this – I wish I had died."

When I left the ICU, I was transferred to the traumatology service of the Virgen de las Nieves Hospital in Granada. While there, one day I heard the doctors telling my family that I suffered from a very rare condition called Locked-In Syndrome. This meant that I was locked inside my own body, and the only thing working properly was my head. They said I wouldn't improve, and that my family should start looking for a place where I could receive life-long assistance. I felt sick hearing this, and I think that was what gave me the push to say to myself, "I'm going to fight tooth and nail against this horrible condition and prove doctors wrong about me. This illness is very stubborn, but they don't know that I am even more so." Tears, asking "why," and lamenting being too young for my life to end like this were of no use.

During the first month, I was completely immobile. I could only move my eyelids a little bit, but my gaze was lost. I couldn't move anything else; I was fed through a nasogastric tube, had a hole in my throat with a breathing tube, and I remember being surrounded by pillows on all sides because even my head had to be propped. The situation was devastating, and I was extremely depressed. That's how I spent the first month, trying to come to terms with the drastic change in my life; but it was difficult not to lose my sanity, because I understood everything that was said around me, yet no one tried to interact with me or address me a word.

So I said to myself, since I don't have a voice to communicate, I will use the only thing I can: the expressiveness of my eyes and my smile. Thank God, people easily understood me, and I got along well with the persons I encountered in my difficult journey.

After four months of extremely harsh silence, something very curious happened. You see, one day, a family member asked me if I wanted to put a picture of my dog on the wall. They said, "Tell me with one blink if it's yes, and two if it's no." When they saw me blink once, they put their hands on their head and said, "WOW, SHE DOES UNDERSTAND!" And then exclaimed, "What you must be going through, being as active as you've always been and seeing yourself like this!" At that precise moment, they put a piece of paper in front of me with the alphabet, and they would name all the letters. When they got to the letter I wanted, I blinked, and that's how I formed words. It took me some time to learn this system because it was very difficult. I had to listen first, then find a short word that encompassed everything I wanted to say while also paying attention to the letters, and during that time, the other person had to notice my blinking. It was a very slow system, but I had no other choice.

One day, my partner said, "We have to refine this system to make it a little quicker." They presented me with a board on which they had written all the letters of the alphabet. They had divided it into groups like the keys on old cell phones, all arranged in two rows to start the word by saying "up" (top row) or "down" (bottom row). Then they would begin naming, "1" and that group contained the letters A, B, C, D; "2," the letters E, F, G, H; "3," I, J, K, L … and so on, saying the numbers first until I blinked, and then the letters of the chosen number. That way, we communicated more quickly, and after a few months, I had gained incredible mental agility. I memorized the alphabet, and we could even communicate without the board. WHAT A GREAT SATISFACTION!

From there on, I managed to communicate more fluently. They would lift me for a few hours a day and sit me in a wheelchair with pillows under my arms and one behind my head. At first, a physiotherapist would come to my room for an hour every day to exercise my arms and legs until I could sit for more hours, and they could take me down to the hospital gym, where they would work on more parts of my body, such as trunk balance.

The days in the hospital were long, but I organized myself well to make them more entertaining. My partner assigned a caregiver to me on weekdays because she had to work, and my hospital was in another province (Granada), while we lived in Almería. This person kept me company when I didn't have therapy; sometimes she would take me to a park to soak up the sun, and other times she would take me to a playroom near my room. There, we would listen to music and play chess or dominoes with other patients from that floor. She acted as my hands, pointing out each piece, and when she reached the one I wanted to move, I blinked in agreement. That's how we could all play, and most of the time, I would beat them all!

One day, a close friend visited me and gave me a book called *The Secret*. My caregiver read to me a little bit each day. That's when I began to believe in the power of the mind. One morning, I realized that if I concentrated strongly on a finger, it would move slightly. Seeing this reaction motivated me immensely, since I understood that if I made an effort, perhaps I could achieve more. That was my daily routine during the seven long months at the traumatology service of the Virgen de las Nieves Hospital in Granada. I noticed improvements in my body, but they weren't enough for me to stay in that institution.

One day, the management gathered us to say that our therapy with them had ended, and we had to appoint a guardian to take care of me because I was listed as single. My father suffered from senile dementia and barely knew what was happening, and my mother had passed away two years earlier. I was very clear about it; I chose my partner. This enraged my siblings, and while we were at it, we took the opportunity to tell them that we were friends and a couple, which made them even angrier. Then my older brother said, "Well, from now on, let your wife take care of you," and they turned around and left.

Only one sister supported me and stayed with me. I felt as if the entire hospital had collapsed upon me; I was greatly disappointed by my family. We had always been very close, and I fell into a deep depression for a month as I tried to digest this new blow. In such circumstances, my partner talked to her parents, told them that we were a couple, and explained everything that had happened with my family. They didn't hesitate for a moment: they opened their doors to me and welcomed me as another daughter, adapting their house to make me as comfortable as possible. For the first six months, from their village (Alhama de Almería), I went to my rehabilitation sessions at Torrecárdenas Hospital in the capital city [Almería]. I was transported by ambulance and received physiotherapy, occupational therapy, and speech therapy between two and three hours per week of each. And on weekends, I continued exercising in an improvised and makeshift gym that my partner had set up at home.

After several months of receiving both public and private treatment, the time came when the system also discharged us. They recommended that I continue my rehabilitation at a Day Center that was going to open in Almería, and would be a pioneer in acquired brain injury treatment. In the meantime, I continued working at home on my own with all the equipment my partner had prepared for me.

In 2011, I started attending CERNEP [Center for Neuropsychological Assessment and Rehabilitation]. There, they researched brain damage and evaluated us neuropsychologically. It was located at the University of Almería. We had workshops of all kinds (meditation, social skills, music therapy, cognitive stimulation, etc.), and we also had an exceptional physiotherapist who started getting me up on a standing frame: incredible, right? What a wonderful feeling it is to be able to stand up from the wheelchair, look at people in the eyes, and give your butt a rest! There was also a magnificent speech therapist who helped me a lot with the mobility of my mouth, my tongue (imagine, it was completely paralyzed), and my breathing, as I still had a gastric tube and always had my jaw slightly open. In three years, I managed to close my mouth and again take fluids through a straw. During all that time, I could only drink thickened liquids; it was horrible to watch people eat while I couldn't even drink water. And in those three years, we achieved that too. The therapist also started trying to feed me pureed food – what a joy to be able to taste food, it was a delicacy for me – and they removed the tube from my belly. After four long years of silence, I began to articulate something with her help – HALLELUJAH! But my lung capacity was so low that I could barely be heard or understood because with the minimal mobility of my tongue, I could hardly articulate. That speech therapist, and the whole team, helped me a lot physically and psychologically, and I will be forever grateful to them.

I noticed all the small advances I was making with a lot of effort – which were huge for me – and that gave me a tremendous adrenaline rush, and I encouraged myself to continue with my fight. At that time, I was obsessed with walking again. A neuropsychologist who was there grabbed me one day and said, "Don't obsess over regaining what, unfortunately, you have already lost. Focus on the part of your body that is still working, 'your head.' You don't know how important it is. Perhaps in the future, you can write and help other people." What great advice she gave me (and she wasn't wrong). I have to tell her that I am writing, and I'm sure she will be very happy. From that day on, I began to change my mindset, and my personal growth began.

At the same time, there were also some positive changes in my personal life. After three years at the house of my partner's parents, we wanted to become independent and see if we could manage on our own. My partner never gave up; she devoted herself to making sure I lacked nothing and that I was never alone. From day one, she was making devices for me to have a good quality of life. Always pushing me so that I wouldn't lose hope. I was ever more encouraged by the fact that, with so much effort, I was progressing and that, little by little, my body was waking up. I remember that my partner was exhausted every night, day after day. That wasn't a life for anyone, and that's when we realized how much work dependent persons demand.

Until one day, I saw a sparrow land on my window, and I said to myself: I want to fly like that bird, see the world, and be surrounded by people like me. At that moment, I considered moving to a residential facility. The first time I thought about it, I got goosebumps, thinking about the many taboos that had existed around residential facilities in the past. Finally, after researching and considering it a lot, we decided it was the best option, so we applied for a subsidized spot through the Social Services.

In 2010, I was prescribed an electric wheelchair, thanks to my partner who requested it from the rehabilitation therapist. She prescribed it with apprehension because she doubted I could use it. At first, I couldn't reach the joystick, so she put it behind me so that she could steer the wheelchair. We stayed like that for a few months, until she adapted it for me and brought it closer to my hand so that I could drive the wheelchair myself. I went from being completely dependent to being able to move without relying on anyone; the situation was incredible, something unimaginable for me! I felt exhilarated and free.

Do you know what the most difficult barrier for me to break was? Going out for the first few times in a wheelchair and being seen by my friends and acquaintances. It was horrible! The looks of sadness and pity crushed me, along with comments like, "What a pity, so young." I never liked people feeling sorry for me; I don't feel that way. On the contrary, I feel very fortunate to be alive and to have another chance. I intend to make the most of it. That was clear for me almost from the beginning. However, on the other hand, I had to face difficult feelings; I felt embarrassed to interact with people, but as you start out, shame vanishes – there's no other way.

I was given a spot in a residential facility in a town in Cádiz called La Línea de la Concepción, a six-hour drive from where I lived. It suited me to have to go so far away. Do you know what struck me the most as soon as I stepped into the facility? Seeing that they treated me like a normal person, and if your family member signed an open regime, you could go out unaccompanied from 10 am to 11 pm. I was amazed because at home, they overprotected me so much that they didn't let me do anything on my own.

There, I met a fellow resident who was as adventurous as I was. He opened for me the doors of disability and helped me value myself more as a person. He said, "We can do almost anything; we set up our own barriers." By that time, I was already using an electric wheelchair, and he said to me, "From now on, I'll be your hands. When we go shopping, you show with your gaze what you want, and I'll get it for you." I felt free and independent; nothing could stop us. I felt so safe with him that I completely lost my fears. Every day, we went for intrepid undertakings, crossing the border into Gibraltar, and we even started smuggling tobacco! He was my teacher, and I will be eternally grateful to him.

I spent two incredible years in Cádiz, but since it was too far from my partner, and she could only come to see me once a month, I requested a transfer to Almería. I was granted a spot in a town in eastern Almería called Albox, where I spent seven unforgettable years. I had completely lost my fears and trusted myself; I had acquired incredible self-confidence. Since the town was small, I knew it inside out in two days, and I went out by myself to wander the streets. And as I gained more mobility and confidence in my speech, as the years went by, I was heard and understood better and better. This encouraged me to go out and run errands by myself, without depending on anyone and feeling autonomous. I began to be INDEPENDENT AND FREE! I started to let go, and went to the bank. I asked the teller to take my ID from my wallet, told them how much I wanted, and they put the money in my wallet. Seeing how well I managed on my own, I gained ever more assurance. I started going to the supermarket on my own; since I couldn't pick up anything with my hands, as they were (and still are) clenched, I would ask the first person who passed by to get for me what I wanted. Seeing how well I managed on my own, I gained more self-trust every day. I went shopping, to pubs to watch football (I love it – I'm a Barcelona fan), to concerts, to flea markets; in short, I signed up for every event. I thought, "Who would have thought, who saw me in the past;" and I told myself, "As long as I can, I'm going to enjoy life because I've spent enough time stuck in the four walls of a hospital room."

There I spent some wonderful years, I felt FREE AND INDEPENDENT. But also went through tough times like the COVID pandemic, which I will never forget. In 2020, fate threw another hurdle in my path: I was diagnosed with breast cancer. I wanted to die! I said to myself, "Damn! What wrong have I done to deserve this?" And do you know what was the worst part? Getting the news behind the bars of the courtyard, without a family member's shoulder to cry on and release my anger. I felt a huge drop; I thought, "After all I've been through, just when I was enjoying life, another blow." When I felt down, do you know how I bounced back? By setting myself a new challenge! My psychologist, seeing me so sad, told me, "The first thing you need to do is give cancer a name." I named it "Bartolo." Now, she said, you're going to fight against it with all your might, and tell your people not to ask you every day how you are doing; that way, you don't sustain it. That's what I did, and it worked great for me; nobody nagged me. I passed on information only when I felt it was appropriate and had news. My roommate, seeing me so sad, dedicated to me a song by Pastora Soler called "Amigas" (Friends). It made me cry to listen to it, because I saw myself so reflected in it, expressing exactly how I felt at that moment. Then it gave me a tremendous adrenaline rush. I recommend it to all those who go through this ordeal; personally, it helped me a lot.

The first time I went to the oncologist, I said to myself, "I'm not going to stay in a corner of my room crying and cursing my bad luck; I'm going to fight once more." It's been almost four years now, and I feel great. I'm still here, the usual troublemaker!

Because of distance to my home, I requested a transfer to a residence in the capital of Almería. In 2022, I was given a subsidized spot at FAAM [Spanish acronym of the Almería Federation of Associations of Persons with Disability], the best one by far and the most comprehensive, with innovative machines, a heated pool, and incredible professionals. Here, 80 percent of the staff have some type of disability; every day they give me life lessons and strength. I think if they can work with their limitations, I can too. What struck me the most when I entered was the great human and close treatment by all the staff. We are like a big family, and I live very comfortable here; I feel very loved, and this has become my true family, the one that lives with me every day. Each of us expresses ourselves in our own way, but we all understand each other. Every day I feel more grateful to have gone to a residence, to live with people like me. That's priceless, I assure you. At first, I thought my illness was the worst in the world. Now I know I was wrong. I've been living in residential facilities for eleven years and have seen all kinds of diseases, each worse than the last. I think, How lucky I am to have a clear mind! And I live in a five-star hotel with full board.

Here in the capital, I've gained a lot in quality of life, outings, and I'm 15 minutes away from my partner, who comes to see me every Sunday. She's happy to see me happy and how I'm navigating life. Every day I speak better and louder, with professional help, but largely due to my stubbornness and desire to progress.

In the physiotherapy gym, we have a machine called ERIGO PRO, it's a robotic bed with which I train standing up, while simulating walking by moving my legs. I personally love it.

In the occupational therapy room, I work on my upper limbs and autonomy. We have a machine called ARMEO SPRING, where I exercise arm mobility by playing games on a screen. The machine assists my movement, allowing me to adjust the gravity and arm joint I want to work on, while blocking the movement of the other joints.

Thanks to scientific research and the outstanding professionalism of my speech therapist, I currently receive Transcranial Direct Current Stimulation (TDCS). It's a non-invasive treatment that uses a very weak direct current that passes through the skull to reach the brain and acts via two electrodes. It produces a modification of the membrane potential that stimulates or inhibits the transmission of information. It has helped me greatly improve my concentration and mental agility. Likewise, my therapist obtained for me an Augmentative and Alternative Communication (AAC) system; it consists of a tablet adapted with an eye tracker that allows me to communicate by voice and manage all my apps.

Do you know why I am like this and have such positive and persistent attitude? When I hit rock bottom, I look back and get sick just thinking about it: "Oh my God, if I hadn't made any progress and had stayed in bed!" It turns my stomach to think about it (given how bad I've had it), and I draw strength from the depths of my soul; that encourages me to keep moving forward without stopping for a second. I am very aware that if I stop, I lose everything in a few days, considering how hard it is for me to maintain mobility by grinding myself every day from 8 am to 7 pm. I thought I had seen it all, but I have some fabulous professionals here; I have a speech therapist, psychologist, occupational therapist, physiotherapist, plus an electric bicycle on which I ride 15 km daily. I organize my days to do a little of everything, and keep my mind occupied to avoid losing it and not get overwhelmed by any activity.

I have been living in residential facilities for eleven years, and I have grown a lot internally; I value the truly important things much more. I have gained a lot of patience. Who would have imagined that eleven years ago, when I was an embodiment of self-centered anxiety? Currently, I think:

- First about my partner. I love her so much because she has shown me beyond doubt what true unconditional love is, and I don't want to see her alone with the cat. Now, I'm the one encouraging her to find a partner and enjoy life as she deserves. I see that she is doing very well now, and I love that. Every day I am happier here, and feel loved by everyone. I am getting better, and increasingly enjoy life; and she, in turn, is very proud to see me so happy.
- Every day I feel more fortunate to have a clear mind. In this world of disability, it's a luxury. Is my body messed up? Yes. And so what? I don't mind not being able to walk: I have wheels to move!

- From where I am, I encourage those who share the same condition as me, LIS, to appreciate and understand that amidst the bad, we can feel very privileged to have the best-kept treasure: OUR MIND. We just have to set our minds to it and soar.
- Today, I feel very comfortable with myself: IF YOU WANT, YOU CAN. I attest to the importance of a POSITIVE ATTITUDE AND PERSEVER-ANCE, and most of all, of having A GREAT MORAL SUPPORT that pulls so you don't sink.
- My partner and I have learned in these years to worry only about ourselves and the people who genuinely love us. I feel very fortunate to have her by my side.
- With regard to my siblings and family: writing this chapter of my life has helped me heal the wounds that were festering inside me. If when I needed them most, they turned their backs on me, now I couldn't care less. They're the ones missing out on spending time with me; I am worth a lot more.
- Doctors always paint a very bleak picture of the future, but they don't know that we have the best medicine: POSITIVE ENERGY. It is up to us to make an effort to fight and have a desire to overcome. That way, pro-gress can be achieved, I can attest to it.
- After suffering from cancer and surviving, I think that seeing the dawn of a new day is a gift for me, and I don't make long-term plans. I enjoy everything to the fullest and live in the moment.
- For someone with no education, I am amazed at how well I write. This is new to me, and it is something I have acquired in recent years. I no longer feel trapped in my own body. I have managed to step outside of it, TO BE INDEPENDENT, and communicate with my own VOICE with a lot of courage. Incredible, isn't it?! I'm living a dream I don't want to wake up from.
- I have had the great fortune of encountering fantastic professionals who have paved the way for me. And mostly due to my great attitude of over-coming obstacles, not to falter in the tireless struggle to move forward in my recovery.
- I am very, very proud of myself, of everything I have achieved with so much effort; it has borne fruit. In conclusion, I like the current Paqui Vil-legas more than the previous one.

I hope that everyone who reads this chapter of my life gets a shot of adren-aline and faces the future with more optimism. I will feel very happy if that happens.

And finally, I would like to say to all the neuropsychologists who are re-searching LIS that I'm delighted to offer myself to try out any new develop-ments that may arise in the future.

Here are my two mottos:

LIVE LIFE (FOR IT ENDS), BE HAPPY, LOVE UNCONDITIONALLY,
AND DON'T FORGET TO HAVE A TOUCH OF MADNESS
and:
THE ONLY IMPOSSIBLE THING IS THE ONE YOU DON'T TRY.

This is my personal email address <supersilla18@gmail.com>, in case anyone wants to contact me, and feels I can help them. I offer myself happily.

I provide you with a photograph taken at the beginning of my story, with the sequelae suffered after the stroke, so you can see with your own eyes the state I was in. And also, a recent image of me, so you can understand that with effort and perseverance, gratifying rewards are obtained.

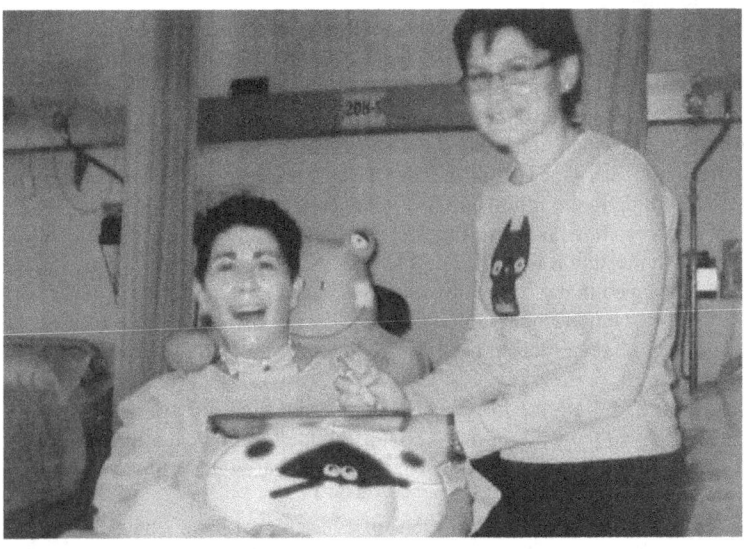

Figure 13.1 In February 2009, after 4 months of suffering a stroke, which left me completely paralyzed, I began to wake up my body. I had a cannula in my trachea to be able to breathe, and a gastric tube to feed me. Surrounded by pillows to support my body, even my head had to be propped. And I couldn't close my mouth. I communicated with a slate, and with the blinking of my eyes.

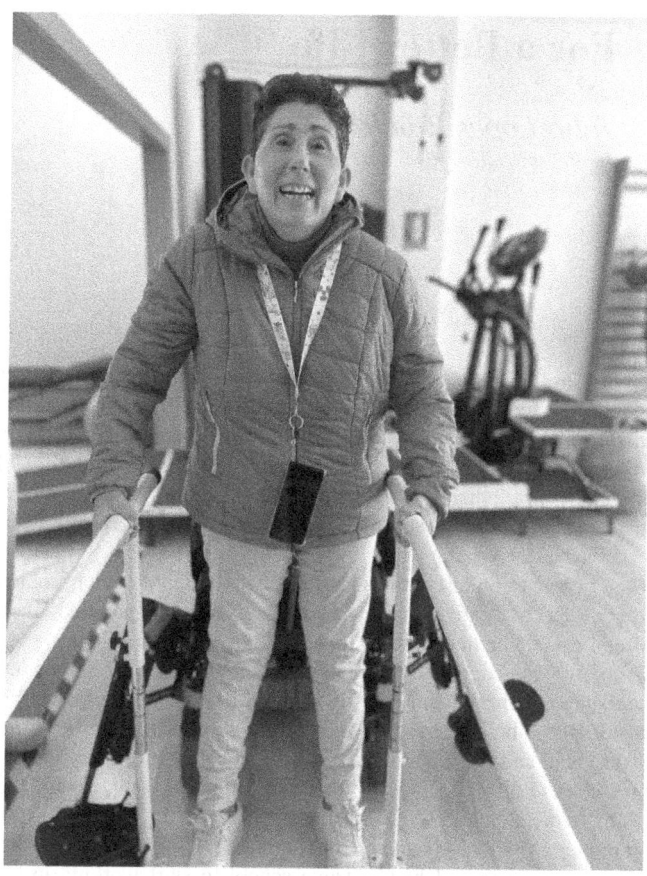

Figure 13.2 Here I am now, in August 2024. Today I feed myself by mouth, communicate with my own voice, and operate my cell phone, iPad and electric
wheelchair by myself. So, you can see a lot of effort and perseverance
can lead to gratifying rewards. The main thing is to have positive energy.

14 For a Better Life

Julio Lopes Ribeiro

I was born in 1971 in a very modest little village in the north of Portugal, the youngest of five brothers and sisters. After my mother died of breast cancer when I was just sixteen months old, my father remarried a woman with a manifest "emotional deficiency "particularly towards me and my siblings. Unfortunately, my father also developed the same lack of affection towards us. Of course, this was not at all the case with the child born of this union a few years later.

When I came to France at the age of thirteen to join my older brother, who himself had left our native country a few years earlier to join his lover, now his wife, it was in the hope of a better life.

Given my young age when I arrived in France, I was a schoolboy learning the language; I learnt it mainly on weekends when I accompanied my brother, who worked as a butcher in the markets for a very friendly boss. At first, all I did was clean and tidy up, pack the meat and sometimes carry the customers' purchases to their cars. As the customers often gave me tips and the boss always gave me a small bill at the end of the weekend, I had a tidy sum of pocket money, which motivated me to continue.

When I was sixteen, I had to leave school to start working in housing renovation. I worked in the building trade during the week and continued in the butcher's shop at the weekends. As I gradually got involved in preparing the meat and selling it, what started out as a small bill became a fully-fledged income.

I learnt the trade on my own, both in butchery and construction, and when I was eighteen I became independent. While it's true that I worked hard and earned a good living, I also spent a lot of money.

A Turning Point

I continued in this vein, but having stopped working in the markets and lost my weekday job, I moved back in with my brother, during which time I worked in a variety of precarious jobs. On a beautiful morning in the summer of 1993, a month before my twenty-second birthday, I got up and, despite the

DOI: 10.4324/9781003464181-14

summer temperature, took a hot bath before going out for a coffee in the bar next door. After drinking my coffee I felt my muscles stiffen and my vision blur. I went out for a walk but it was getting harder and harder to bend my knees, so I went back to the bar to sit down but I couldn't bend my legs. I felt worse and worse and could see myself going. I vaguely heard the bar owner calling the firefighter. He must have also called my brother because I heard his voice before passing out.

This was followed by a deep coma lasting a fortnight and a long period of delirium where nightmares and reality merged. It was impossible to know when I was asleep or awake, as everything was a nightmare. In some I was fighting hard in a ruined city, hiding in its basements from an invisible enemy. In others, I was alone, shouting but no one could hear me, and shadows moved around me whispering who knows what, which wasn't much more reassuring. It seemed like an eternity when in fact it only lasted just over a fortnight. But there was a shadow who regularly came and held my hand. His presence soothed me, and I felt through that firm, reassuring hand that nothing could happen to me in his presence.

And then, after a long time, these shadows gradually took on human form. I began to perceive faces and the whispers became understandable. The most dreadful of my nightmares was in fact reality.

No matter how hard I tried, no matter how much I screamed, I was trapped in my body, completely immobile and mute. As for the shadows and whispers, they were the nursing staff chatting during my treatments and the shadow whose presence soothed me was my brother who came every day to keep me company for quite a while. The whispers that accompanied him were the TV that he turned on when he arrived. And as he didn't turn it off when he left, I had a presence, at least until one of the nurses decided to turn it off, thinking that no one was watching and thus condemning me to the sole company of my distressing thoughts.

The doctors did try to communicate with me, but as my eyes were immobile and blinking was automatic, I had no way of signalling my presence. They were well aware of my presence following the various tests carried out (CT scan, MRI, etc.), but communication was impossible at that stage. I'd had a serious ischaemic stroke. A stroke can be ischaemic or haemorrhagic: ischaemic, where an artery becomes blocked, preventing the brain from being properly irrigated; haemorrhagic, where an artery ruptures, causing a haemorrhage with the same more or less devastating effects. As someone who never does things by halves, I was of course entitled to the most devastating one.

One day I was transferred to another hospital where there was no television in the intensive care unit, but the staff often spoke to me despite the fact that I didn't answer. In my room, it was often a parade; in addition to care and physiotherapy, the nurse had to regularly supply and monitor the proper functioning of the various machines. There was one with a tube through a hole in my throat to help me breathe, one with a tube through a hole in my stomach to send liquid to feed me, one to monitor my heartbeat and others that were doing I don't know what else. In short, I was pierced everywhere and surrounded by numerous machines. The malfunctioning of some of which would cause my "immediate departure", something I obviously wished for many, many times.

One fine day, one of the nurses, who was particularly attentive, arrived in my room with a television. I have no idea where she found it or how she managed to get it into intensive care, but I was no longer alone. My face was certainly beginning to be a little expressive and, as she was so attentive, she was able to perceive it. In short, she had to give instructions, as I was always left with the television on (except sometimes when I was asleep).

Then the doctors gradually removed the machines one after the other until all that was left was the one that fed me. It was the most psychologically disturbing of all because I used to dream of a rare steak with lots of French fries, a ham and butter sandwich or fried eggs. Instead, all I got was this brownish liquid that went straight to my stomach. Because of the paralysis of my jaws (among other things), it was impossible to feed myself orally.

After almost six months in intensive care, I was ready to go to a re-education and rehabilitation centre. The doctors seemed quite pleased with themselves, but I was a little less so, as my future life seemed very bleak and I couldn't really see what they were going to be able to "habilitate", given that I was totally immobile. I then convinced myself that it was impossible for me to live long in these conditions and that I was bound to "go" soon, all I had to do was wait.

It was around February 1994 that I joined this centre where everything was based on re-education and rehabilitation. There was a whole team of physiotherapists, occupational therapists, speech therapists and even psychologists, but what was I going to do with a psychologist given that I couldn't communicate? As the doctors once told me, I had Locked-in Syndrome (LIS), which meant absolutely nothing to me and, unfortunately, not only to me, even the doctors seemed to be a bit lost. Even though we now know more about it, the evolution of LIS is unpredictable and varies greatly from one person to another. The vast majority of cases are caused by strokes of the brain stem. I have to admit that the days at this centre were very busy. For instance, the physiotherapist was putting me on a table to move my limbs in all directions and then strapping me in firmly before putting the table in an upright position where I stayed for almost an hour. I liked staying in this position because then I could look out over the whole room and see the team of physiotherapists working around all these bodies bruised by life's accidents, each one more serious than the last. The occupational therapist was subtly trying to accentuate the slightest small movement likely to be exploited. The speech therapist was making me make ugly faces in order to wake up the slightest facial muscle useful for speech. I barely had time to stay in my room so the machine could slowly feed me.

The occupational therapist soon prepared a chart with the whole alphabet for me, to try to get me to communicate. Although it took a while at first, I soon got the blinking under control and even made a few small head movements, so I was able to communicate. She would show me the letters one after the other and when she reached the letter she wanted, I would blink to let her know.

In this way, the letters became words, which in turn became sentences. Having said that, I personally found this system far too slow and tedious, and it irritated the hell out of me; I soon gave up on it. So the occupational therapist had to find another way for me to communicate and continue doing my "exercises". It wasn't just a question of getting me to communicate; her idea was much broader (I realised this later). So she found an electronic typewriter and designed me a helmet with a rod (a unicorn); this enabled me to type on the keys of the machine. For me, the task was less irritating because I could see the letters being printed on the paper, one after the other, but for her, it made it more difficult. As I didn't move my head from side to side, she had to move the machine left and right so that I could reach the letter I wanted. A secretary types an average of seventy words a minute. I could almost do the same but in an hour.

One morning, they kindly decided to shampoo my hair. The caregiver put me in a chair and led me into the bathroom, where he placed me in front of the washbasin and lowered my head.

There was a mirror in front of the bathroom sink and before he lowered my head I caught a fleeting glimpse of someone I didn't recognise, which intrigued me enormously. When he'd finished shampooing, he put me back in the chair and I had plenty of time to observe. I got the shock of my life: it was really me, fifteen or twenty kilos lighter. Normally I wasn't very well-covered, but this time I was a shadow of my former self.

In spite of everything, I continued to do what was asked of me but with relative detachment, passing on all my discomfort to the occupational therapist, as she was the person I was most often in contact with. One day, one of the doctors came into the room and, seeing us "fighting" with the typewriter, offered us his old computer that he had used during his studies. It was an imposing screen with a hard drive with a very, very limited memory, but it had the advantage of a removable keyboard that was easier to move around than the imposing typewriter.

Little by little, with a lot of exercise, my head started to turn to either side, very slightly at first but soon enough that the occupational therapist no longer needed to move the keyboard, she put it on a stand and let me write relatively independently. I still needed help, but very occasionally. The occupational therapist was the only person who thought she could improve my living conditions; neither the doctors nor any other caregiver believed in it and even less so myself.

That's when she told me about the possibility of driving an electric wheelchair, thanks to the slight movements of my head. Despite my misgivings, she made an appointment with some sellers to let me try one out. She was right: with a control placed just in front of my chin, I was able to move around. Also, as it was a standing chair, they could stand me up anywhere at any time.

Although there was a good atmosphere in the physiotherapy room, there wasn't much variety. The occupational therapist, convinced of her good idea, set about ordering the chair without delay (with my participation, of course), informing me of the importance of standing up.

It is very important for a completely immobile person to be able to stand regularly, for good blood circulation, for example. This is very important because it only takes prolonged poor circulation for small skin redness to appear and things can then very quickly degenerate into bedsores. The bedsore is a truly horrible thing, the flesh literally rots. I was able to see one on my roommate, it had taken all his buttocks, then a pestilential smell emanated from it. I think the nurse deliberately made sure that I could see because when she finished the treatment and dressed him, she came to see me to explain. She told me that it is very painful, complicated to treat and takes a long time to heal, this gentleman was "lucky" not to have sensitivity in this area. Well, "luck" not really since he couldn't feel the warning pain either.

By "luck" I have kept the sensitivity intact throughout my body (a particularity of LIS) and thanks to the vertical chair I would be able to get up as soon as I feel the slightest pain and thus relieve the point of support by restoring blood circulation.

In short, here I was a few months later with a chair adapted to my needs that I operated myself. The beginnings were rather difficult, because of my very limited head movements. As soon as I moved a few millimetres in the chair, I had a lot of trouble reaching the controls and needed help. Of course, it was the occupational therapist I asked to help me with this task; patiently, she adjusted the control I don't know how many times a day. Fortunately, my movements gradually improved and I needed her help less and less.

One day, or rather one evening, just as I was expecting the nurse to arrive to connect the machine that was feeding me, a nurse arrived with a steaming plate of porridge. She pulled me up from the head of the bed to a sitting position and gently began to spoon the porridge into my mouth.

I couldn't tell you what it was, but I found it delicious. It was the only food I'd had in my mouth for almost two whole years; the many grimaces the speech therapist had been making at me for months had finally paid off. Not really in the area I'd hoped (speech), but it was thanks to her hard work that I was able to master opening and closing my jaw as well as slight tongue movements. Of course, they didn't stop feeding me through a stomach tube all of a sudden; it was a gradual process until I was able to eat by mouth alone. Even so, I had to keep the tube in place to get water. Liquids tend to go into my respiratory tract, which makes me cough a lot.

Despite the fact that the physiotherapist had no results, I was now able to communicate, move around and eat. Given that the centre couldn't expect any further progress in the short term, they started looking for another place where I could live and continue to slowly develop my achievements.

My brother then offered to host me. He started converting his garage into a bedroom/bathroom. In 1995, without much enthusiasm, I moved in with him, because as far as I was concerned, all I would be doing there was waiting for an imminent departure (although I was having more and more difficulty convincing myself of that). My brother worked all the time and was hardly ever at home. His wife was already looking after their three young children, so there was little time left for her to devote to me. Apart from the physiotherapist, speech therapist and care assistant who came to see me to do exercises and care, I spent my days in front of the television and didn't communicate much, even though my brother had bought me a computer. Every day I became more withdrawn and thoughts of my imminent "departure" became more and more present.

Moving Towards a Better Life

One day in the summer of 1996, my brother decided to send me on holiday to an adapted centre in the south of France. I think the holiday was mainly for him and his family, because I admit that I wasn't very easy to live with at the time; they needed to breathe and take a step back.

After a long and winding train journey with its not always convenient changes, we arrived at the holiday centre, where I was dropped off. The staff there were very kind and attentive, and I went on a few outings to parks and other places. I had a lot of trouble getting my wheelchair to move because I hadn't done any exercise for months, I didn't leave the house and I didn't use the computer. I spent a month there without any means of communicating, which suited me just fine as I had no desire to do so at the time.

However, that stay changed my life completely. I met a totally paralysed and mute thirty-something who was being wheeled around in an armchair like a package. I later learned that this person was born disabled, which made me realise that it was entirely possible that I would have to live in these conditions for a long time. It was around thirty-five degrees and yet an icy shiver ran through my entire body. That man seemed not to be aware of his state which was not my case at all. He probably doesn't have the capacity to do otherwise, but I can move around alone, I can communicate and I have about average intellectual capacity (well, I think).

When I came back from this stay, the possibility that I might live for a long time in these conditions haunted me constantly and it took me a long time to come to terms with the idea. One day, I saw a man with LIS on the TV news who had just published a book. Even though he only moved one eyelid, he dictated his book letter by letter using a chart like the one the occupational therapist had made for me. I can only imagine the amount of patience he had to have, because after two sentences I was at the end of my tether, whereas he wrote dozens of pages! He had energy to spare.

In short, after having digested this awareness, I started to open up a little to break out of the isolation into which I was inexorably sinking more and more every day. I started reading the Association des Paralysés de France (APF) magazine that I received every month and talking to the speech therapist who always came to help me with the exercises, as well as my brother and his wife. It was then that I felt the need and desire to go and live in an adapted home like the one featured in that magazine.

If I'm going to live, in spite of everything, I might as well improve my living conditions and if I continue to stay with my brother, I have little chance of achieving a better life. I spoke to him about it and although he was a bit offended, he took the necessary steps. His vexation was completely understandable. He had modified his house to accommodate me in good conditions and not even three years later I'm asking to leave.

LIS acts like a tsunami, devastating everything in its path - the life of the person affected, of course, but also the lives of their family and friends. Relatives think they can deal with it on their own and are full of goodwill, but it's better to leave it to the professionals, at least at first. The LIS sufferer is in great psychological distress and inflicts his suffering and rage on all those around him. It is therefore preferable that those around him should not be their relatives but professionals who are trained and used to dealing with them.

Settling into Independence

Finally!

When I asked to move out of my brother's house, I was probably thinking only of my own well-being, but with hindsight I think it was the best thing to do, both for me and for him and his family.

The following summer (1997) I went to spend a month in an APF establishment to test whether life there would suit me. This time, of course, I brought my computer so that I could communicate. There were different disabilities in the establishment but I was the only LIS person, I went out a few times and the establishment was quite large with long corridors where I could practice driving the wheelchair. I also had a lot of conversations with residents and caregivers, which meant that during my stay I did a lot of writing and my head movements were very much in demand.

I really enjoyed life there, with offices staffed by nurses, caregivers, cleaners, a linen maid, a cook, physiotherapists, an occupational therapist, all the necessary equipment and someone to look after the wheelchairs and the premises (plumbing, electricity, painting, etc.), not forgetting the entertainers who organised outings and activities according to the wishes and desires of the residents. There was also a large dining room, as well as a number of smaller rooms that could be used for a variety of purposes. It was quite a change from my little room in my brother's house. When I returned to my brother's house, all I could think about was: "When can I move in?"

In the APF magazine that I received monthly, there was a "letters from readers" section, I started replying and, strangely enough, I liked writing. It's true that at school I really liked French, but my level of studies was not very high.

I had little chance of finding a new career in writing. Then one day, I received a letter informing me that a place had become available and that I could join the establishment at the beginning of December, i.e., one month later (the first of December 1997). I was very excited at the idea of living there and, reading the magazine I noticed that one of my responses had been published which, in addition to making me very happy, gave me a certain confidence in the "future". I was confident that a new life was opening up to me. Well, it probably was not what we could have dreamed of, but it turns out that my future looked less bad than the doctors' predictions.

The day finally arrived! The room I moved into looked more like a studio than a simple room you'd expect to find in a medical-social establishment. It had to be at least twenty-five square metres.

There was a toilet with a large washbasin (in the establishment there were several large communal bathrooms) and a kitchenette with a sink. Of course, this wasn't really for cooking, but more for having a fridge and a work surface for a microwave, a coffee machine or similar.

There was a medical bed and a built-in cupboard, and the rest was up to each person to decorate as they wished. As far as I was concerned, I had to keep as much space as possible so that I could move around freely with my wheelchair, which I still didn't control very well. I didn't want the room too cluttered. I had just moved into a real living space; not into a place of care but a place where I could live.

Barely having time to familiarise myself with life in an establishment, I continued to read the association's magazine and respond to readers' letters. Since I had been published once, I was hopeful of being published again, so I applied myself very seriously. Then one day, a new response, then another and it even became regular. It amused me to write these little articles and it made me very proud that they were published. When I wrote, I didn't think about anything else and even forgot about my situation.

One day I learned that the LIS person who had written the book with just the blinking of an eyelid had also created an association, the Association du Locked-In Syndrome (ALIS). I made contact, more out of curiosity than anything else. I met many other LIS people as well as dedicated and caring people who were there to help us.

The atmosphere there was warm and I must say that it was very appreciated. It is also thanks to the help of the ALIS association that I was able to acquire, in 2000, a complete set of IT equipment: a desktop computer equipped with a virtual keyboard on the screen and of an infrared system that, thanks to a patch stuck on my glasses or forehead, allowed me, by moving my head, to direct the computer mouse and click using a timed click. Using such a system requires great precision, which unfortunately not all LIS people possess. Some need more complex and expensive equipment controlled by eye movements. I also acquired a laptop computer equipped with the same system which I could carry everywhere and use to express myself. I was thus equipped to subscribe to the Internet and have direct and easy access to news, reading, music, films and, above all, emails to send my articles, which were now published regularly in the magazine.

In the establishment good care was taken of the residents who were encouraged to become as independent as possible. Together we found an external speech therapist (the sessions were quickly cut short due to lack of results) and a nurse. I used to go to the drugstore myself to get the equipment I needed, first accompanied by a caregiver but quickly on my own. Just like the dentist I regularly saw in a hospital. I ordered transportation by email and went there independently. She was a very nice dentist who took care of the administration herself. As for the appointment, she gave it to me one after the other.

One day they fitted my bedroom door and one of the lifts with a remote-controlled electrical system, then fitted me with an environmental control system. An environment control is a bit like a universal remote control but a little more sophisticated; you can connect anything that can be re- motely controlled. I could control: the TV, the radio, the light, the call system the establishment was equipped with (like in hospitals), the door to my room and the elevator. This means that once I was seated in my chair, I was relatively independent. I could be on my computer and decide to watch TV, or I could leave my room, take the elevator and go to the drug store, or just take a walk outside. Well, it's true that alone I couldn't go too far away so I stayed nearby.

I then made friends with a resident who was much more independent than me (Aude) and sometimes we went for walks together. Since she was very independent, she could help me in case of problems, which allowed me to travel around the city and the parks in complete safety. It's really thanks to her that I gained some confidence. Occasionally we met outside and I didn't mind taking a long journey alone through the city that I knew by heart. Without our outings together I would never have had the confidence to dare to go far away alone in a wheelchair.

Finally I took advantage of the fact that the staff were busy elsewhere to get used to a certain level of autonomy. They were present in the establishment if necessary but otherwise, everyone lived their life as they saw fit.

After living in the establishment without problems for about seven years, I began to have desires elsewhere. Especially since I was eating better and better, it wasn't yet the rare steak or fried eggs that I dreamed of but I was slowly getting closer. As for drinking, I took gelled water by mouth. Gelled water is simply water that is heated with gelatin; as it cools, it takes on a compact texture and thus avoiding pulmonary aspiration. It's frankly not very good and having this tube permanently stuck in my stomach was psychologically very disturbing for me. Removing it became vital. I now have a powder made from modified corn starch, without taste or odour and which, mixed with any cold or hot liquid, thickens it in two minutes. This allows me to drink a small glass from time to time: wine, whiskey, champagne or others… Well, drinking a glass of good wine and eating a kind of wine-flavoured compote is not at all the same thing, but when you have no other choice, it's still pleasant.

The lack of staff was more and more and it was becoming difficult to find support. Even getting help with meals was becoming complicated. Whereas before it was very rare for a caregiver to help two totally dependent people at the same time, little by little it became the norm. The establishment became a factory and the caregivers were working on the assembly line. They had no choice. There were fifty-two residents to take care of and the teams were always understaffed. The staff no longer had time to chat or discuss things and no spontaneous outings were possible. Even those planned for a long time were often cancelled at the last minute due to a lack of accompanying staff. In addition, writing my little articles which were now published very regularly, no longer pleased me as much as before. I continued just out of habit but without much enthusiasm, so I gradually stopped doing it. Even though life in an institution suited me for years and allowed me to gain confidence and independence, it became more and more burdensome. I told the general delegate of ALIS (Véronique) about my discomfort and she assured me that it was now possible to move into an apartment and live alone with twenty-four hour assistance.

To achieve this, I began by contacting my legal guardian telling her of my desire to live independently in an apartment in the city. I was then confronted with his formal and categorical opposition, deeming this option far too dangerous. I took a few days to digest the news before writing directly to the guardianship judge who appointed a doctor to assess my ability to live independently. She was a very friendly lady, helpful and attentive, with whom I spoke for more than two hours.

I later received, as did my guardian, a summons to hear his verdict; not only did she give me the green light to live alone in an apartment but she also reduced the protective measure which then became curatorship instead of guardianship. A guardian can manage your life as she sees fit, while the curator is required to do so with you.

This is how Véronique Christian (an ALIS volunteer), the now curator and others took care, not only of applying for social housing but also of all the administrative side which opened up the possibility for me. I had the right to assistance from carers twenty-four hours a day for all acts of daily life, as well as various other forms of assistance. Barely a year later I was offered a two-room apartment in a quiet location; when I visited it, I found it a little small but the landlord was willing for me to make modifications. *So that was it.*

With the valuable and wise suggestions of Carole, the occupational therapist who has become a friend, we completely redesigned the apartment. To be able to move around with my chair, we removed some partitions and moved others. Véronique transformed herself into a site manager with whom I was sometimes very impatient. The small two-room apartment where I could barely move when the furniture was in place had become a spacious, very functional studio where I could easily move around. The downside was that since I needed 24-hour assistance, the caregiver had to sleep in the living room. As we had to remove the partition which separated it from the bedroom, there was only a simple curtain between us.

Yet, I lived in this proximity for almost 5 years before I was offered a magnificent three-room apartment in a very good location where I have lived since 2012. It's certainly not a palace but I'm comfortable there, I have a bedroom for myself, one for the carers, a bathroom, a living room and a kitchen which both open onto a balcony where I can enjoy the sun. It's not huge but I have everything I need and I feel very good there. I get up and go to bed when I want, I go where I want when I want, I eat what I want and above all I can finally eat "my steak with fries and my fried eggs" (among other things). I can finally live for myself without worrying about whether I will have someone to accompany me and help me.

It is still incredible to me, the unsuspected capacity for adaptation of human beings. At the very beginning I didn't even understand the idea that we could live in these conditions and today I find myself appreciating my life as it is. It's also true that it has evolved enormously since the day when, in that hospital room, I became aware of the extent of the damage and my catastrophic state. I am far from being the only one to appreciate my life as it is because most LIS people live their condition well despite everything.

I must admit that I was very lucky to have met the right people at the right time who supported me, helped me, put up with me often but above all, constantly encouraged me.

My plan is to take full advantage of every pleasant moment that life is willing to grant me and if I have to "leave" tomorrow or in ten years, so be it, but I'm not in a big hurry anymore.

15 Black Dog

Dawn Faizey Webster

28th June 2003 is not a date I will easily forget! It was two weeks all but one day since my son had been born in an emergency caesarean section. Although I didn't feel a thing I was aware of everything that was going on, and I did hear the surgeon say that he was stitching me up like a Cornish Pastie to which I voiced my displeasure. I remember listening for a cry for signs of life from Alexander to make sure that he was OK, after all he was only 26 weeks old at that point and I was not going to be allowed to go down to see him until the next day. Fortunately I did hear that all important cry so I could relax momentarily. Simon, my husband, was allowed to go and see him and came back with a card adorned with tiny hand and footprints declaring that it was a "Happy Father's Day" on Sunday June 15, 2003, now Alexander's birthday.

I spent the following week in hospital, settling in as best a routine as can be achieved in a week, each day revolving around visiting the 1 lb 8 oz, 11" long Alexander that was now in an incubator in the special baby unit of Stoke-on-Trent Maternity Hospital. After waking up at around 7:30am breakfast was a self-service affair which consisted of some of the best hot buttered toast that I had ever popped out of a toaster, followed by a nerve-wracking trip in the lift down to neonatal. I can remember the heart in the mouth, butterflies in the stomach feeling of heading into neonatal to find out what kind of a night Alexander had passed.

After sitting with him for an hour I would leave the unit and go back up to my room in maternity, envious of the mothers with their babies with them, blissfully unaware of what the very near future had in store for me.

It was during this week that the infamous black dog incident occurred. Whilst in Stoke Maternity my husband, Simon, had been visiting me every day, arriving at around midday and leaving late evening. It was on one of these evening journeys that, when driving through Colwich, out of the corner of his eye he saw a dark shape dart across in front of the car, so he braced himself for the inevitable thud that was bound to follow. As expected, it came immediately after, and he stopped the car as although he didn't know what it

DOI: 10.4324/9781003464181-15

was at the time he just knew it was big. Fortunately he saw what he could then identify as a large black dog continue on his journey to one of the houses on the opposite side of the road.

On telling me this the following morning I can clearly remember thinking to myself how they say that a black dog is an evil omen (or perhaps I was thinking of the Hound of the Baskervilles, it doesn't really matter now) so I was beside myself worrying that it foretold of some calamitous event befalling Alexander, having little or no concern that it foretold of anything happening to me. How wrong I was!

All I wanted for that week was to get home but everything wasn't going back to normal after the birth of Alexander as they said it would, and they were reluctant to discharge me but after much persuasion and agreement to continue with the medication for high blood pressure they let me go. It was a bittersweet homecoming though as something was missing, I wasn't bringing my baby home with me, but I assured myself that I would see him every day just as if I was still in hospital. I didn't know at the time that my husband had other plans and that I was on countdown to a life changing event. That evening after a fish and chip dinner I learnt that my husband didn't intend to visit Alexander daily because of the cost of the fuel, which was about to be the least of my worries.

Every morning of that week I would phone neonatal for an update on Alexander and how he faired through the night and boy did I dread making that call in case it was bad news, but it had to be done. In the afternoon we would visit him at neonatal and sit with the tiny Alexander in his incubator, it was during one of these visits that the funny turns started, I can only describe it as suddenly feeling extremely dizzy with a very heavy head and neck pain and extreme difficulty in focusing my right eye and walking in a straight line. It was like being drunk and having a hangover at the same time. Eventually it would go off, although each episode was a bit more severe and longer lasting than the previous one so by Friday I had confined myself to the settee and I was having trouble focusing on the episode of *Quincy MD* that I was watching. I am not sure if I fell asleep or simply went unconscious but I opened my eyes to find Simon right in front of me saying that we needed to go to the shop and that he had phoned the midwife about these funny turns that I kept having. She thought I was probably low in iron because of the blood I had lost during the caesarean, and she would write up a prescription for me to collect from the doctors. If I had thought about it, I would have known that this could not have been the case because of the high blood pressure that I was suffering, but I made the mistake of trusting the professionals rather than my own thoughts.

We got the prescription along with a bar of chocolate and we decided on broccoli with dinner, all with the aim of increasing my iron levels and putting an end to what I still called my dizzy spells. All the time this was going on and from even before Alexander was born I had been having a pain in the back of my neck that had warranted the occasional use of paracetamol, but this had simply been put down to a crick in the neck and was never really given serious consideration no matter how much I complained about it.

This was on Friday evening 27th June, the following morning Simon had already arranged to get an early train up to Doncaster (I think) to collect his new motorbike as he was getting rid of the virtually brand-new BMW that we had bought for two up touring as now we were three. I awoke early to the strangest sensation ever like feeling dizzy, drunk, leaden headed and hungover at the same time and not being in full control of my right side as it was hard to keep my hand still to dial the telephone. My speech was slurred and it was quite clear to me (and everyone who saw me) that I had had a stroke, Simon's answer to this was to call my parents and get out of there as soon as possible. In hindsight it could be seen as putting his new motorbike before his wife but at the time he was the last person I wanted around when I felt so bad and he had a motorbike on his mind.

When my parents arrived, they took one look at me and dialled 999 immediately, unable to disguise their disbelief that Simon had simply upped and left when I was so clearly seriously ill. Fortunately it didn't take the ambulance long to arrive and they bundled me onto their chair, swaddled me in blankets and whipped me away to Stafford hospital A & E. Little did I know that it was the last time I would ever see my house or my beloved cats.

On reaching A & E, I was taken straight into a cubicle and transferred onto a bed to start the long wait that characterises A & E on a Saturday morning. I estimated that I arrived at around 6 am and by lunchtime still nothing had happened and I was starving hungry and desperate for the toilet when finally a doctor came in and decided to do a blood test. Unfortunately he had already decided to take it from the groin area so I said I must go to the loo first otherwise when the doctor came near me.... well you can guess the rest! Luckily a sympathetic nursing sister brought me a bed pan and basically told the doctor that he wasn't doing anything until I had been to the toilet.

After that I was whisked away for a CT scan (the MRI scanner was broken and with it being the weekend there was no one available to fix it) which showed that I had no bleeds on the brain, which was all they were looking for at the time although I had been complaining about the pain in the back of my neck for around 2.5+ weeks. They continued to say that this bore no relation to my possible stroke and even gave me some paracetamol for the pain even though I had told them that I had had difficulty in swallowing since that morning.

By this time it was late afternoon and I had been moved onto a general ward and hooked up to a drip of drugs to reduce my blood pressure. To continue with the barrage of tests to understand quite what was going on, two junior doctors came to give me a lumber puncture in order to test my spinal fluid, so I duly curled up on my side while they had their first attempt. They failed, they tried again and failed, tried and failed, tried and failed, tried and failed, tried and failed, tried and failed, tried and failed, until after trying one final time and failing they admitted defeat and left.

By then the evening visiting had started and my parents had been home, collected my husband (who they had found polishing his motorbike without a care in the world considering his wife and severely premature son were seriously ill in hospital) whom they were most displeased with. I had started foaming at the mouth like something rabid which I can only attribute to my reduced ability to swallow.

When visiting ended I settled down for a sleep, initially I attempted to watch the TV but as there was only the one small screen to the whole ward and the angle it was facing rendered it very difficult to see and hear especially with the other patients gossiping away to each other.

I couldn't say what time it was, all I remember is that the general ward lights were still on so it couldn't have been that late but I suddenly felt really weird, like I had been hit over the head with a sledge hammer. I rang for the nurse who came straight away for a change and I could feel myself slipping into unconsciousness. Just before I went I managed to blurt out to the nurse "I don't feel very well", then everything went black.

I came to at some unknown time immediately aware that I wasn't able to speak and I couldn't move the right side of my body, although I was still in control of the left side as I can remember hooking my toes of my left foot around the back of my right ankle to straighten my right leg. I was also acutely aware of the fact that I could see double and the pain in the back of my neck had got much more intense as I can remember pointing to my neck to indicate this to my brother who had stayed with me all night. Apparently as it was a Saturday, there were no senior doctors in Stafford hospital, so they had to speak to a consultant, who was in theatre so we had to wait for him to phone back, to discover that I had a blood clot in the back of my neck that was affecting my brain and I needed to have anticoagulants as soon as possible.

I was to be transferred to Stoke-on-Trent Hospital that night/early morning, and as they were preparing for the move I slipped back into unconsciousness. I was only told later that for the move I was taken off the anticoagulant drip because from then on I was not fully conscious for around two weeks, but I kind of drifted in a strange semiconscious state when I was aware of things happening as if they were in a dream, like having my hair washed whilst thinking I was an Iraqi soldier! I also have a hazy recollection of friends coming to visit me although it was more like a "Star Wars" moment in that I felt their presence rather than remember seeing them.

It was after about two weeks that I started to feel properly conscious, and I could properly say that I was awake. The problem was that no one else realised this and the movement down one side that I had in Stafford hospital before the transfer had now completely gone so I had no way of making any one aware that I was fully conscious. The doctors had a very scientific test

– they would hold my hand and say, "squeeze my hand if you can hear me" and I would think "love to mate but that's not going to happen!" I remember I didn't feel very frustrated by this but more annoyed at their stupidity. Eventually it was my husband that noticed when he held a magazine up for me to read that my eyes were following the words and therefore, I must be conscious. Unfortunately the doctors would not believe this and said that I wouldn't be conscious for weeks if not months yet.

It was at this point that my brother had the blinking good idea of blinking as a form of communication and he got me to look up for yes and down for no, he then started going through the full alphabet stopping at the letter I blinked on:

a b c d blink
a b c d e f g h I j k l m n o blink
a b c d e f g blink

and there it was, my first word in blink speak, dog. The excitement that it created in my family was immense, you would have thought that I had recited the complete works of Shakespeare verbatim!

My sister-in-law must have spent the whole of that evening thinking of ways to improve the alphabet system so that whoever I was talking to would not need to go through the whole alphabet every time and she came up with the four-block system, which simply involves choosing the block in which the letter appears followed by the required letter.

| A B C D | H I J |
E F G	K L M
N O P	T U V W
Q R S	X Y Z

so now to spell out a word like dog would be:

A blink
a b c d blink
A H N blink
n o blink
A blink
a b c d e f g blink

and at last someone had found the key to letting me out. At last I could tell them that my legs were really painful, and please could someone rub them before I went crazy! I really thought it must have been evident in my face,

I didn't realise that I was completely expressionless at the time and it was several weeks if not months before I regained movement to the left side of my face but unfortunately the right side of my face never has regained any movement whatever. The only good thing about this (glass half full and all that) is the complete lack of wrinkles as if I had had a full facial Botox.

This led to the second major medical disaster, as in the loss of my right eye – initially this was caused by unfortunate neglect on behalf of the hospital, and I didn't even sue! While I was in the High Dependency Unit, they put drops in my eye daily as it didn't close properly and was quite dry, when I moved into a normal ward once I was known to be fully conscious, they were not aware of this and no drops were given. Consequently my retina became very badly damaged, and I had about four different types of antibiotics in my eye, initially every fifteen minutes and eventually saving my sight, albeit very cloudy and blurred through a tremendously scarred retina. All the absolutely amazing care that I received from one particular ophthalmologist was undone as I caught an eye infection and virtually overnight my eyeball went soft and I finally lost my eye. At that point I was so used to not seeing through it properly that the loss of sight by now hardly bothered me by then.

I was now in the Haywood Rehabilitation Hospital, and I had been there for about five months by this point, everyone said, "oh they will work you really hard at the Haywood, you will be begging them to stop". I couldn't wait for it and five months later I was still waiting for something to happen. Intensive physiotherapy meant a once a week stand in a standing frame and that was only because my parents went and fought for me to get one hour a week as a set time, and this is how it went on for the fifteen months that I was there. I believe that if my mother hadn't asked about me coming home, this situation would have simply continued as it was.

After two years in hospital, on the 17th of July 2005 I finally came out for good to a hospital bed in my parents' dining room temporarily until their garage was converted into a separate bedroom with a wet room for me. Care was provided from the local social services team with three calls a day, with my parents filling in the gaps with passive movements and other details such as cleaning my teeth.

There have been many changes through the years, starting with the decision that all clients requiring permanent full-time care had to move to a private care provider as social services were doing short-term care only. As a friend of mine was starting up her own care company, I decided to go with them and one of the social services team came with me. Unfortunately as the company grew the original care concept fell by the wayside and personal care became rather rushed and impersonal as I turned into profit rather than a person.

Just at this time COVID struck and everyone was having their own struggles with the illness, lock down and its associated issues, when the most devastating event took place. My mom passed away from a non-COVID related illness. This led to my deepest darkest depression from which I could see no escape, I desperately felt pointless and hopeless with nothing in my future to look forward to but days of the same, regular care and being unable to do anything for myself, no use to anyone and just a burden to the rest of my family.

The turning point was when I applied for my own Personal Health Budget and set about employing my own care team. Finally I felt I had a positive purpose in life, I was an employer and I actually felt like I had carers who cared because they actually looked after me and only me. Also because I now had care throughout the day from those who could drive my mobility car, I was finally able to go out in the week when I wanted to, and this really made a huge difference to my quality of life. One of the main factors now in my life is going on holiday and I have found that people in other countries are much more welcoming and helpful to the disabled rather than fearful of approach as they seem to be here.

This seems a quick way to skip over the last twenty years but that is how it seems to me to have gone. I can never say that I have accepted what happened to me or that I ever wish that it hadn't, I can't say that I don't look at others with envy that I am not up and walking about and having a "normal" life, and I am so very thankful for my son being at my side always, as well as the love and care of my family and the carers that I now think of more as friends. It's precisely because of this that I have completed a bachelor's degree, a master's degree and hopefully soon to be PhD. Together with Tracey Gibb (who was also living with LIS) and neuroscientist, Shannan Keen, we initiated the first ever annual webinar on Locked-in Syndrome, which continues now to be fully administered by Shannan as I was not able to give the time required due to the work involved in my PhD. This now brings us to the present day where I am living day by day, writing this and not looking too far into the future other than planning holidays for the coming year.

16 Conclusion

Shannan Keen

This book has allowed us to gain insight into the lives and achievements of twelve people, in different areas of the world, living with LiS, being unable to express yourself or move any part of your body; the fear of suddenly being surrounded by people not realising that you are alert yet unable to communicate. Their resilience, patience, despair, frustration, happiness, perseverance and appreciation of life shine through in each of their chapters. As their writing has revealed, anyone can have a life-changing event. These individual accounts have shown us how they have each adjusted, coped with and, in many instances, conquered some of the enormous challenges that LiS brings.

As we have read, the diagnosis of LiS comes after much pain, suffering and intense frustration. While Locked-in Syndrome is not common, the impact of a person with LiS upon their family, loved ones, friends, workplace and community can be enormous. People with LiS require extensive hospital services for diagnosis, management and therapy, adaptive equipment, home modifications, respite care, and social and financial support. Many of these services are largely dependent on state or federal funding. Through wider knowledge, such as this book, it is hoped that, by getting better information on LiS, we can argue more convincingly for better funding of hospitals, clinics, therapists, technological communication and mobility devices, diagnostic and research services to improve the care and outlook for these vulnerable people.

Three of the chapters enabled readers to learn about some of the outstanding professional people in technology, science and medicine in this field. It is a privilege to hear about their ground-breaking work for, and with, those who are living locked-in. They have each outlined for us plans and aspirations for the future. It is of vital importance to accurately test and assess the cognitive abilities of all people who are unable to express themselves following accident, disease or injury. These damaged people are unable to communicate yet are fully aware of everything that is going on around them. Medical science is making remarkable progress with diagnostic methods and treatments. Neuroscientists, medical practitioners, nursing staff, neurotherapists, communication and IT experts all need to work hard to continue to improve diagnostic methods. In particular, which cognitive assessment protocols are

DOI: 10.4324/9781003464181-16

being applied and which of those are empirically proven to be accurate, which treatments patients are receiving and which of those therapeutic regimes are offering the most beneficial outcomes.

We have read of the intense frustration of being locked-in, with medical staff, nurses, carers or family chatting and ignoring the 'patient'. Some countries appear to be better than others at identifying those who are locked-in. More effort must be put into learning from those nations that are doing these things the best. More work must go into training medical practitioners to do their utmost to identify signs that the person is locked-in. Regional and national governments in all countries must recognise the importance of funding to enable people with LiS to live the fullest and most autonomous lives possible.

Time and patience are of the greatest importance in evaluating people with LiS as it is extremely tiring for them to attempt to respond with only eye movement or blinking. It is essential that those with LiS play an active role in decision-making processes regarding their rehabilitation. Many of the people who have contributed to this book have stated that they felt 'lucky' that those around them realised that they were fully cognisant. 'Luck' should not come into it.

Devices to aid in communication and other assistive technologies have proven beneficial as well as allowing individuals to become active members of society. They strive for independence. Eye-tracking devices permit affected individuals to use a computer with artificial voice, control their environment, surf on the internet and send emails. As our communication expert states in his chapter, it is important to recognise the transformative power of these tools, not only in restoring communication, but also in rekindling a sense of identity and participation in work, study, social and family life. However, as another of our LiS contributors notes, the difficulty of non-verbal language is that it is a language without gestures or alternative communication systems such as sounds or expressions. It is composed solely of eye movements. She, and each of our LiS authors, speak of the great difficulty in conveying information via a spelling board, eye-tracking and computer devices; these are open to interpretation or misinterpretation by the person who is being talked to and they don't allow for shrugs or winks, smiles, grunts, chuckles or grimaces. The subtle shades of prosody and tone are lost. Apart from the ever present 'emojis', they are bereft of emotional expression. As that contributor said, it is a language that bruises all LiS people.

In rare cases, some individuals have recovered limited motor abilities. Those who recover some motor control in hand or head can use this to communicate with a computer and sometimes control their wheelchair. Improvements are frustratingly slow. The person with LiS and their carer must work hard and be extremely patient. As more than one of our LiS authors have said, some feats seem unachievable at first; persistence and patience is required for every gain.

As we are all aware, the past couple of decades have seen an explosion of technology and artificial intelligence in communication and assistive technology. Computer programmes allow anyone to study for a degree, learn another language, create art or compose music, as some of our LiS contributors have successfully achieved. Artificial intelligence (AI) is already able to help us construct sentences, correct spelling and grammar, translate languages and can give a 'voice' to those left without the means of speech. That is just the beginning. Within the foreseeable future, AI will continue to build on these capabilities.

Brain-computer interfaces (BCI) have the potential to restore a voice to someone who has lost the ability to speak, with expressivity, speed and effortlessness as in natural speech. Already multiple research institutions are working on proof-of-concept demonstrations of brain-computer technology. In this book, we have read about one of the successful implantations of BCI into a person with LiS, both from the perspective of the LiS person herself and from one of the team who designed and implanted the device. In future, this technology can become an option for patients with Locked-in Syndrome, enabling them to 'speak' and express themselves without the need to 'type' every word.

International collaborations have been made possible in part due to computers and interconnectivity. The sharing of information and the collaborative work of teams from many areas of the world are enabling new strategies and creating novel solutions. The willingness of professionals to work with those in disparate fields opens our minds to the potential offered by others in broadening our horizons and enabling wonderful achievements.

As our LiS authors have demonstrated, their lives can be full of achievements and joy. We encourage you to share this book in order to help others to understand more about this condition, to learn from the remarkable abilities of those working with, or living with, Locked-in Syndrome. It would be marvellous to think that some of those reading these words will be inspired to dedicate their own lives to pushing forward the boundaries of medicine, science and technology in the drive to continue to improve diagnostic and treatment methods, communication devices and all that is currently, and will in the future, improve and make life easier for people living with LiS.

Index

Page numbers in *italics* indicate an illustration/photograph